Praise for *The Intuition* ~~~~

If your self-worth is tied to your achievements and service to others, yet your own deepest dreams go unfulfilled, you have found the right book. Positive, light-filled, and healing, this masterfully written spiritual guidebook shows you how to find more Joy and less stress so that you can live a joy-filled and purposeful life.

—Gay Grant, author of *Destination Unknown*;
former Maine State Representative

I love the number of small gems hidden throughout, the reframing of common problems in a way that exemplifies a lifetime of learning and growth.

—Raynor Large, Certified Business Advisor

Sirois will be the first to say that life can be a messy work in progress, and the pursuit of Joy can be difficult. The simple but powerful concepts she shares are the result of decades of putting thoughts to paper, of reflecting and teaching as life unfolds. *The Intuition Manual* is an invaluable guide for self-care, self-reflection, going within, and celebrating your Greatness.

—Collette Sosnowy, PhD in psychology;
researcher and former journalist

The Intuition Manual

~

A Guide Toward Mastery
of a Key Self-Care Habit

BOOK 1

D. Anne Sirois

Hazel
Marie's
GARDEN

The Intuition Manual, Book 1
2024 © D. Anne Sirois
ISBN 978-0-9849229-6-3

Original cover art, "Blossoming in the Joy," by D. Anne Sirois
Photography by Petra Jayne Sullivan
Cover and book design by Lindy Gifford, Manifest Identity
Genie Dailey, editor
Hazel Marie's Garden, publisher
www.hazelmariesgarden.com

Note: The acronym *FOG*—Fear, Obligation, Guilt—was popularized by Susan Forward, PhD, and Donna Frazier in their book, *Emotional Blackmail.*

The content of *The Intuition Manual, Book 1,* is based solely on the author's personal experiences and is not a substitute for professional advice in the reader's life pursuits.

Contents

A 1000-Peace Puzzle . . . 1

Hazel Marie and Me . . . 11

FOG . . . 19

Our Body Boundaries . . . 29

Coming All the Way Home . . . 43

Follow the Path of Joy's Persistence . . . 51

Daily Peace Rises and Sets Within You . . . 71

Guided Journaling . . . 99

You Are Not Bound by the Hands of Time . . . 109

Ascensions . . . 125

SWAT Teams . . . 135

Greatness Is in the Eye of the Beholder . . . 149

The Joy of Knowing . . 161

Wrap Us in the Gift of Your Presence . . . 173

A 1000-Peace Puzzle

You matter.

What you say matters.

How you feel matters, what you do matters, what you value matters. You are not a black hole of matter, destined to live with…"it" doesn't matter.

You do not have to give your time and energy to people to whom you do not matter. You do not have to give your Self up to another person, to the point of your pain, *or beyond*, for a cause that does not include *you*…in the matter.

You can trust your Self to find the people you matter to. You can use your intuition to help you decipher the matters that are important to you. You can trust your Voice to figure out how to *share* with others the things that matter the most to you.

You can rely on your inner spirit to help you understand *why* you do what you desire to do, and *who* you desire it to matter to. And to include your Self in the matter because your peace and Joy also matter.

It takes some time and energy to develop a life *knowing* all this. It takes a consistent connection to a Greater Power System to learn, master, and *know* you reside in a world where you can live a *whole* life, where you don't have to live a life in 1000 disconnected pieces.

It takes a deep connection with a Voice that teaches you that you, putting those pieces together and honoring how you fit into the Greater Good, *matter.*

How you experience peace matters. How you express your Self matters. How you experience Joy matters. How you encounter the truth matters. How your imagination is embraced matters. How you live, love, learn, and leave a legacy matters. These are all crucial pieces to include in the Greater Good puzzle.

In my life, I've experienced relationships where people did not care about me or champion what mattered to me. In some cases, I was just a disposable means for their ends. In some relationships, I was just an "it." Instead of a living, breathing spirit inside of me—the other "I" in the relationship with them—I was (unbeknownst to me) an invisible servant of *their* "we."

Within these relationships, I was seduced by their "we" thinking, mistakenly assuming my equitable turn at inclusion would eventually come.

What mattered to me—slowly, piece by piece, disappeared from my life. But the *relationship* mattered to me, and that word *we* kept me tethered to *their* me, until I realized their "we" would ultimately mostly just include *them.*

After a point, I decided *I* mattered enough to exit their "we" and enter into all kinds of relationships where "we" fully included me.

During those hollow "we" relationships, little by little, I contributed more and more of my energy toward their desires. And over time, I found myself devalued, and the spirit breathing inside of me slowly ceased to be fully alive in the black hole of their "right now."

When I perpetually found myself in a shared space where I became their "it," when I found myself in their implied and disguised "Shhh—be silent" (aka, your preference doesn't matter *right now*) over time, I lost the strength of *my* Voice.

When they perpetually implied and disguised "Shhh—don't be selfish" (aka, your dreams aren't a priority *right now*) over time, I lost the value of *my* time and energy.

When they perpetually implied and disguised "Shhh—let go of your needs" (aka, mine are the ones that are most urgent *right now)* over time, I lost the balance of *my* power.

There was a repeating pattern, as they implied and disguised "Shhh—don't think of what's missing in your life" (aka, just live with "it") and over time, I lost the evolution of *my* life.

There were times that I spent being routinely scared shh-itless, in the service of another's "right now." And it took me a while to realize that the perpetual sacrificing of my peace for their "right nows"… resulted in my never-ending wait for the perpetual shh-it to end…until I just finally put an end to my participation in the relationships.

I also stopped planting my Voice in people whose opinions and actions implied, then disguised, that because I did not matter to *them*…I did not matter, *period.* I stopped trying to live within an endlessly oppressive environment where life was frequently viewed as "shh-it," according to *them.*

I exited the negativity in perpetuity and began redirecting my time and energy toward digging up long-buried bones of what I knew to be true and beautiful about my Self. I extricated my Self from the shh-itty environment I was in and unearthed my buried soul.

I went into my mental backyard and dug up the lost pieces of me, one by one, and assembled them, peace by peace, into a spiritual skeleton held together with the strongest spine I never knew I had.

I evolved a whole new picture of my Self and grew a whole new vision of what was possible for me.

Then I found new ground to plant long-abandoned dreams in. I spread fresh clean fertilizer and grew a whole new life to house the spirit that was breathing holy fire inside of me. I changed the internal radio station from believing I was only entitled to a barren land of inability to remembering that I *own* an abundant land of capability.

I changed my tune to one that guided me to share my life with those in whom I *know* my opinion matters. I relearned how to make *me* matter, by removing the *shh* in "shh-it." And instead, I embraced my Self...transcending "it" to a whole, connected, united *spir*-it.

When I refer to my spirit, I mean my Voice, my intuition, my "gut telling me" to go toward, to do only, to feel deepest...Joy. I'm referring to my spirit as in the Joy within my Greater Power System directing my preferences, my values, my dreams...until *I'm* satisfied.

The state of "it" wasn't worth much until I figured out what the health of my spirit was worth to *me*...until I figured out what my job was, in regard to the possibilities for my life.

So I started respecting and honoring and paying attention to the condition of my spirit, and first raising *my* belief that I was valuable. And with time and energy spent positively and proactively progressing my actions from abstract potentials to concrete finishes, I began to believe in more of who I could be and deliver more of what I could do.

I began raising my Self with a belief in a Greater Power System that included me in the Greater Good—growing my Self in my own Voice, planting my Self in my own soil, feeding my Self with my own sun, watering my Self under my own rain...trusting my own Joy, sprouting my own blossoms, multiplying my own garden of desire, sunning in my own results.

I have worked hard to answer the question, "What might one need to raise one's Self to full glory, with a Voice one can *trust*?"

What might one need to truly raise one's spirit with a courageous belief in one's own *power*? And not secretly, blindingly, and repeatedly be tearing "it" down, wearing "it" down, killing "it" softly, with, "Shhh-it, what *you* want just doesn't matter."

I started journaling and writing down the answers that became my strongest Voice in life. I continued digging for honest answers to questions that I could regularly gut-check my Joy with.

Like…do you feel as if you owe someone the sacrifice of your life in order to be in a Joy-filled relationship with them? Is there someone you are still in "debt" to, and that no matter what you do, you still "owe" them? Do you have an idea of when and how they will get paid off, to *your* satisfaction?

Are you driving yourself to arrive somewhere important to you? Is your primary drive a god-driven dream, but your deepest satisfaction is to no avail? Is your work fueled with unreasonable demands on your god-given talents, and you're "successful" if your efforts are only on sale? Is your self-care packed with god-awful strings attached to "it," with your progress hampered down to the last detail?

Are you a train going so fast down the line, so focused on the tracks laid before you…that you risk your spirit derailing? How much energy and power do you have to get to *your* finish line? Do you have a GPS (a Greater Power System) that you can trust to guide you and help you arrive at the destination *you* desire most?

Where is your "I've arrived" located? Who or what challenges your efforts to arrive? Are your arrivals crowded out with other people's forced priorities on your life?

What would your life look and smell and taste and sound and feel like when you finally sit in the moments you arrive in, and you then know you *have a life*? Where do you envision your Self traveling off to next?

If your spirit is inundated with powerless relational collusion or societal noise pollution, it can be incredibly hard to take some time to *sit* once in a while and get some freaking peace, so you can siphon off the stress and feed your deepest cravings for Joy. It can be hard to make the time and own your energy to get to the end of your life *satisfied.*

It might be hard to stay on top of shh-it. Modern life is insanely crowded with decisions, schedules, and duties. You might be like a dog with a bone, digging with a singular focus for that elusive *knowing* that will comfort you in your choices.

If your life has gone by without you living with what you know in your "bones" is what's right and best for you, maybe the time has arrived to bring that Voice, that spirit living deep inside of you…back to life.

Your whispering spirit might be bugging you to get to the bottom of your dissatisfaction, imploring you to get to the marrow of your bones. Maybe your bones have been buried long enough, and now is the time to dig that Joy in your spirit *up.*

You'll have to carve out time and energy to resurrect your hidden Joys, buried deep within those bones. If you're willing, go ahead and excavate every last one of those bones with as much self-care as you can muster.

Just remember, when you're hungry for completion, when you're thirsty for fulfillment, but you can't take breaks or rest for very long (because you're committed *right now*), understand that you *can* get everything that's inside of you out, just not all at once.

But don't sacrifice. Surrender to the directions of your Voice, and don't sacrifice your Self with choices that don't include you.

And know that you'll need help with raising your spirit from a child in need to a fully autonomous adult *meeting* your needs. You'll have to ask your spiritual SWAT teams, to help you find your way, to help you locate where all your Joy resides. You'll have to frequently exercise trust in your GPS to help you unearth the pieces you left behind in the hustle and bustle of the daily world of growing your Self *up*.

You might need to make some changes in your life, so you have more freedom to choose. You might need to lean on someone for longer than expected to help you fit the crucial pieces of you back into your life. You might need to ask for help to figure out all your right moves and next steps.

With time, finding your pieces will get easier and easier and your Joy will grow. Over time, the pieces you've dug up will come together effortlessly to form a whole new life. You'll process every one of those bones and receive training beyond what you think or feel and learn what you *know*. You'll climb your way out from under any landslides of worthlessness and shh-it with new beliefs and a newfound power to choose.

To start with, try choosing to believe it's not a mistake to *desire*—all the pieces that are inside of you, all the pieces that you find yourself missing with every bone in your body. To desire all the pieces that now guide you to *finish* your dreams—*knowing* that you have what you need.

Choose to believe you can exercise your will to move forward long enough to get closure with what's missing. Choose to believe you can live your life lean enough to make ample room for your ambition.

Choose to believe your heart will touch others deeply enough with the consistent efforts of your mission. Choose to believe you can share your Self easily enough to feed those in need with compassion. Choose to believe you can balance your self-care enough beside others that are your relations.

Choose to believe that you will experience meaningful results enough to do what you came here to do—raise you and your spirit, in unison.

Choose to believe you've already *earned* your way to right here and right *now*…over and over and over. Choose to believe you can return "home"—to your spirit, to your body, to your mind, to your soul… again and again and again.

Choose to believe *you* are a spectacular, wonder-filled…hot-air balloon full of Awe. Choose to believe you are loving enough, you are caring enough, capable…yes, even super human cap*able.*

You are more than just this day of frustration, despair, or confusion. You are more than okay…just the way you are. You are okay to be *more* than who you are, to write your story just the way *you* like it.

You are okay, not just to write your story, but to *right* your story— to right your wrongs and to get life right for you. You are okay to straighten your life tall and good and true; then mortar it with the *right* building blocks, built with compassion and gratitude. Then you can share that rightness of you with everyone you desire to.

Your "right" might not be everyone else's right. It might be their left. It might be their wrong. It might be their not right now.

You might have a unique way of healing. You might have an exceptional way of helping. And you definitely have a GPS that can guide you to a life of distinction—your very own Waze.

It's okay to include your Voice at the dinner table conversation, gracefully. It's okay to desire an abundant life that speaks to you, passionately. It's okay to live a life that includes the best of you, spiritually. It's okay to work and rest and play, meaningfully. And it's okay to share the bounty of your life with those you wish, endlessly.

With your GPS guiding you, if the worst happens, you will be strong enough to survive it. But when the *best* happens, you'll know you are worthy enough to *deserve* it.

All that peace generated in putting your puzzle together—and to be at peace with all those pieces, takes an entire lifetime to assemble.

You *will* get enough done, and you *will* experience enough satisfaction with your spirit trained in Joy. You *will* gain the power to emerge from the shh-it fully alive and whole, as you live a life that matters to you. You *will* end up progressing not only your own Joy, but through *your* spirit lighting the way for others to enjoy, too.

Hazel Marie and Me

This book was born over the course of my life as I grew my spirit up from a girl with a Voice inside of her to a woman with the connection to her Voice, *mastered*.

As part of this mastery, I have this belief that there's a guiding hand in my life. And I realize it was passed down to me from my mother. It wasn't so much what she taught; it was how she lived.

I grew up with the transformation of her Self from an indoctrinated Christian to an experiential spiritualist. She washed her family and closest friends continuously with her faith, her conviction, her *certainty* that a Greater Power System (her GPS) existed at every moment of the day to assist her and us.

It was through her personal experiences that we witnessed her Joy and awe at the power she felt when she was "dialed in" to Spirit. She poured comfort over each of us, every time we were in the presence of her being with her GPS. Her daily example of how she grew to stay so connected to Joy with her spirit and to those she loved nourished us. She provided a steady drip of empowerment and real hope, filling our pots to overflowing with comfort.

As I grew older, she became the life-affirming and hope-filled water I copiously drank from. When she was connected and you needed her at the deepest level, she was spiritual water on rock, gently, persistently, and *powerfully* eroding your fears, guiding you to leave behind only the strength of all the beauty in you. You could feel the warmth of her spiritual core healing you. Within the power of her spirit, you learned from her Joy.

She was so encouraging with the certainty of her *knowing*. Her actions originated from her strong beliefs honed from a lifetime of mastery with her Voice. She was my garden tender in that way—constantly feeding me, encouraging me to grow and be and learn and…to just grab onto Joy with all of my heart. The words that regularly came out of her mouth were frequently enthusiastically reassuring.

She was often my example of a bridge we could create for ourselves to the upper world. She was the rock I leaned on. An example of how a rock could be—should be—with *stones* of assurance in her Self. Sometimes she would sit quietly, and you could see her just breathing in the presence of her GPS right in front of you. You wouldn't disturb her, you just sat still with her…in her *knowing*.

She wasn't without imperfection; she was human. Frail sometimes, too strong sometimes, full of fear sometimes.

I grew up with mostly idyllic childhood experiences mixed with a few overpowering ones. She was firm in her ways. I went to church with her faithfully and frequently. I stayed out of "trouble." I helped with chores around the house and just played at growing up.

I am the youngest of five, so I spent a lot of my free time with family, and a few friends. I had been hard-of-hearing since I was three, so sometimes the school and social experiences were disappointingly hard for me to enjoy. I did (and still do) much better in smaller groups of conversation.

I was an above-average student, despite my hearing handicap. I stayed out of team sports that relied on hearing my teammates well and instead, I created art, I ice skated, I cheered, and I attended school dances. I fished, camped, and hung out with the clan, and our lives revolved around the family sawmill business and tons of creative endeavors.

By the time I was thirteen, my dad died, and it was just me and Mum. She took over running the sawmill with two of my brothers. When I was in high school, she was lonely and anxious about her last chick flying the coop, and we fought about it. But two months after I graduated, at age 17, I began hairdressing school with her full support.

My mother was a very shrewd, imaginative, and crafty woman, who was almost a daily example of innovation and creativity and generosity. I grew up being encouraged to use my imagination all the time.

At 21, with my mother's help, I opened my first salon. When I was 27, my mother was determined to secure my future and bought me my first home. At 28 and 30, I had my daughter and son, respectively.

During the years before I had my children, my mother and I occasionally argued, off and on. She wanted me to spend time with her to offset her lingering loneliness, which served only to distance the young and "independent" me.

I had to fight to reset new boundaries with her as a young adult, but after a time, she adjusted to her empty nest and reset her Self. After a little while, I had had enough psychological air with which I could breathe to reset *my* Self, and I once again enjoyed her company immensely.

Over the course of the years, we grew very close, enjoying our mutual love of all things family-related, sharing our arts and crafts, and honing our spiritual minds together. I saw her almost daily in some stretches, when she wasn't jetting off to Canada to go see her brothers and sisters. She was number twelve out of fifteen!

She lived independently in a beautiful home she had built just a few miles from all of us kids.

When I was 40 (the same age my mother was when I was born), my mother discovered she had six months to live. She was extremely organized about preparing for her death. She tidied up her will, had all the funeral arrangements made, and set about selling her house so we kids would not have to deal with it after her passing.

She cleaned out her house, gave away most of its contents, quickly sold the house, and brought the core of her memory-laden possessions with her to an apartment at my home, where she lived out the remainder of her life.

Of these possessions, one of the most important to her was her flowers. She loved many different kinds of flowers and spent most of her life growing and tending to them; so much so that she essentially kept a mini greenhouse of her favorites in her dining room. It was these favorites that she brought with her to set up in her new space at my house.

The remaining days of her life were spent just being present with the family, working on various arts and crafts, and tending to her flowers. As she grew weaker, one by one, she had to let go of each of the projects she was working on. She struggled to hang onto the care of her flowers, but the day finally came when she knew she wouldn't be able to take care of them any longer.

It was on this day that my closest friend, Gay, came to take me out for a break from the caregiving. I was reluctant to leave my mother, but she insisted I go out. She said she was tired and planned to lie down for a nap while I was gone.

Gay and I went out for a while, and when we returned, I found my mother looking particularly joyful. She was sitting in her favorite chair and invited Gay to stay and visit. I couldn't help but notice she was just *glowing*.

We settled in and she excitedly began talking. "Anne, after you left, I sat in this chair looking at all my flowers and getting upset, realizing I had lost the strength to take care of them. And I wasn't ready to let them go. But I was tired, so I went to bed, and I was feeling sad as I fell asleep."

She leaned forward and lowered her voice. "Then I had the most wonderful dream…I was in this garden. And the light was so beautiful. And I saw the most beautiful flowers…in the most amazing colors, as far as the eye could see. Then I heard this Voice speaking to me, telling me, 'Don't worry about your flowers, Hazel…you can let them go. Do you see all *these* flowers? These are for *you*. I have a *garden* here, waiting for you.'"

She paused and started to tear up and shake her head in disbelief. Then she said brokenly, "Can you believe it? There's a garden waiting for me." She paused again and with incredulity, repeated, "There's a garden waiting…for *me*."

She kept saying this with bewilderment, over and over…trying to grasp the dream.

We were all in awe. I looked at Gay and then at my mother…Mum was in tears of disbelief mixed with profound humility and Joy. Gay and I were in tears of heartache—mixed with profound amazement and admiration.

At this point, some family members walked in, and the revelatory moment ended.

But this powerful connection lingered between us. We spent the rest of the afternoon conversing with my mother, basking in her energy and Joy.

As the day wore on, I found myself processing what had happened. I was particularly moved by my mother's dream, but I was surprised at the revelation that this exceptionally wise and strong woman, who had spent many years teaching her loved ones how special and valuable we all were, needed to be reminded of that herself.

This floored me. I was very close to my mother, and I had no idea that she did not see herself in the light *we* all saw her in.

She had spent the better part of her life nurturing an intimacy with her higher power, working daily to create a deeper connection to it.

As she continuously searched for a deeper truth, growing into her wisdom and wholeness, she truly became a master of the spirit. She had this unshakable resolve that there was a guiding hand in her life because she felt so connected to her GPS; her GPS was real to her. It inspired everyone around her, and we all drew strength from that.

My mother's reaction to her dream taught me something very important. It showed me that even the strongest among us sometimes need reminders of our beauty and truth. I realized how powerful a gift this message was to my mother. It didn't matter to her whether we believed her dream was real, or not…*she* experienced it, *she* felt it, and, more importantly, she *believed* in its message.

But the surprising gift of this was that, through her presence, I felt like I was in the presence of something Greater. Through her, I saw the beauty and truth in her through her experience, and I could *feel* the strength of awe planted in her from her GPS.

Before that day, I wouldn't have been able to fully describe to you what beauty and truth sounded like, or looked like, but in that moment, I *knew* it existed beyond a shadow of a doubt. I could hear it speaking to me through my mother as she recounted her dream with such hope and peace. I could see the light of Joy in her as her spirit looked at me through her eyes, when she cried with such humility and gratefulness.

Over the next few days and weeks, through her demeanor, I could see she was still absorbing the comfort, respect, and power contained within this message. Just like the flowers that absorb water and light and the nutrients they need to grow, I could see her rising to accept this gift, blossoming in the understanding that she was, indeed, worthy of this garden.

My mother's dream was a personal milestone for me…the greatness of this intimate moment awakened something in me. It was a pivotal event, because I realized that no matter how strong we all appear to be, we all need to experience Joy in our lives. We all need to hear the words that we are valued, to feel the light of worthiness…to recognize and embrace our own significance in the presence of something Greater. At the deepest level, we all have a need to know that we are really cherished and loved enough, and *feel* seen.

This moment taught me that not only could I seek to embrace this Presence within my own life, but there was just as much power in experiencing it through others.

My mother's dream then became my dream…it became my calling. I found myself on a mission, trying to figure out…how I could help even the strongest among us to remember this glorious power in our lives—to remember the Joy we can utilize to raise our spirit, because I now knew that we all can forget the magnificence of who we can become with Joy *powering* us to greater heights.

I had no idea how this calling would manifest itself, but I knew if I waited…in the right moment, the "how" would reveal itself.

It took some time to learn that my Joy is carved from the life within my spirit and that my spirit comes most alive when I write and teach and paint and entrepreneur and play.

From the steady drip of Joy that I receive from within my guided journals, I am able to continuously chisel the rock of my being, piece by peace, into the art of *me*. And as a result, I take the seeds of that powerful Joy that grows in me, and plant it into other people's gardens—to pay it forward into other people's lives.

And then even more Joy is returned to me.

This book contains the first of many of my most profound journals and the lessons I learned about self-care and raising our spirit. It includes stories of when I stumbled and faltered through my fears and shortcomings on a journey to a greater Joy and self-worth. These are the lessons I teach in my guided journaling courses of when I humbly, haltingly, and daringly, absorb and embrace a greater Presence in my life.

FOG

There is a way to serve others and still serve your Self, while you live, love, learn, and leave a legacy.

There is a way to see clearly through any relationship fog that is abusive to your spirit.

There's a way to drive your Self through any reduced visibility of fear, obligation, and guilt, and emerge in clear and cloudless weather to enjoy your life, to drive and take in all the scenic Joy along the way to your fulfillment.

There's a way to not get lost in any relationships, to not lose your power or your peace in those low-lying, obscuring thick clouds that slow you down, disorient your inner drive, steer you off the road, and scare you away from your dreams.

I found my way through FOG—through fear, obligation, and guilt, with guided journaling and my GPS.

I emerged from some negative relationships with my Joy intact, to resume driving my dreams to my destinations, to guide my dreams and finish them, without being eroded to the point where they were abandoned because of my weather-beaten exhaustion in maintaining unnecessary stressful relationships.

For us to have the spiritual capacity, tenacity, and audacity to shine our Selves out into the world, we need our way forward to be free and clear of unnecessary FOG—to be unburdened of unnecessary fear, obligation, and guilt.

There are foggy people who can obscure our insight and restrict our spiritual visibility. They can disorient our inner compass, confuse our gut instincts, and cloud our intuition.

The fear they dispense can tether us. The obligation they dispense might bother us. The guilt they dispense may fester in us.

There were times when I was afraid to practice self-care—when my needs had to be pushed aside because I had to concentrate *all* my time and energy on driving through excessive FOG.

There were times when I had no choice but to shove my needs aside until I could exit a relationship that had me trapped into choosing between no self-care for me and a "positive" relationship with them, or self-care for me and a negative relationship with them.

There were times I was too exhausted to fight to get included in the Greater Good—when I was forced past my limits of sacrifice, and I couldn't stop the constant assault on my inclusion in Joy.

I became too tired to fight for my self-care and too exhausted to keep the relationships "positive." Having my relationship choices reduced to either me or them, instead of both me *and* them, became impossible choices to make.

I realized it was excessive FOG pressing upon me that blocked me as I drove on the road to more Joy, less stress. So, I buckled up and drove away from the relationships, with my self-worth intact, and I ditched the abuse.

I remembered from my spiritual training that my Greater Power System can see what I cannot, and I just had to listen for the right directions.

It is a dark power that won't let you see far enough to get anywhere near Joy. It is a dangerous power that seeks to make you lose your bearings, sometimes at the risk of your life.

And it is a Greater Power System that gets you the hell out. It is a Greater Power System that keeps the roads clear of abuse.

And it is a Greater Power System that guides you to take the best route to arrive at the place you dream of, full of Joy.

As I said earlier, I was fortunate to be raised within a Greater Power System, with my family and my local church community at the helm of my training.

I was blessed to grow up with such a charismatic, positive group of humans. It wasn't until I was much older that I realized how special these people were.

I was exposed to their healthy view of sacrifice, giving of ourselves and doing good deeds for a Greater Good, that didn't mean we sacrificed our Joy.

And I learned to forgive others, because they taught me our offenders weren't the only ones whose shh-it stunk. We weren't perfect ourselves, so we were morally bound to cut them some slack, but that also meant we were morally bound to forgive our Selves, as well.

My church and family community did a good job of addressing appropriate fears, fulfilling reasonable obligations, and exemplifying healthy guilt that produced light and healing for so many people.

They taught me how to balance my Self with others. The view of the Greater Good that raised me *included* me.

From a social construct, this Greater Good view that I learned steers humanity toward positive, loving, connecting, caring behavior toward others, without losing our Selves in the process.

But when the Greater Good gets bankrupted by negativity in a relationship, when an excessive FOG rolls in that steers us away from our Joy, when the reciprocity in the relationship stops including us, the relationship becomes abusive. The negative relationship can obscure the healthy view…*of all the Joy we deserve.*

The turning of the other cheek becomes quite handy to an intentional abuser who wishes to take advantage of our fogged view, so that what we do for them at the *excessive expense* of our Selves…is *spiritual.*

An empathic and conscientious mind and heart is well aware that everyone makes mistakes. But an intentional abuser's goal is to trick us into believing that our mistakes *always* create more spiritual debt than theirs, for which we must "pay" out of our exhausted bank account.

With an intentional abuser, we can become saddled in a relationship of perpetual debt. They try to make us feel like we're never good enough. They seek to tether us with the promise that with enough good deeds we will *eventually*…be debt-*free.*

Abusive FOG can be an isolated event. But some abusive FOG experiences repeat. Both can have negative energy that can stay with us until we clear it from our spiritual body.

Clearing abusive experiences out of our lives so we can get back to serving the Greater Good requires us to be connected to our Greater Power System to restore us to our own full power.

I used to struggle with balancing my immense creative appetite against the relationships I served.

I was insanely hungry for the beauty and truth I found in all my art forms, but excessive fear, obligations, and guilt robbed me of my peace and freedom as I tried to satisfy my Self with my art.

At first, I didn't know how to curb it other than to write and paint and design and teach and entrepreneur and play, and just get all the torment out of my system and then "make up" for it with binges of serve, serve, serve, to rid my Self of the stress of reciprocity owed in the negative relationships I was in.

After a period of spiritual restoration with my GPS, I was able to rebalance my Self after exiting FOG.

I was able to co-create truly reciprocal relationships where we share normal fears, normal obligations, and normal guilt.

I have found people I can share a lot of who I am with, artistically, entrepreneurially, and spiritually. Within my sharing, I am still driven by my need to serve, but now it includes my Self.

The searching in vain to be "good" enough is over, because I have finally grasped the fact that all of who I am is who I need to be, every single day. And no amount of abusive FOG is going to make me lose any of the pieces of me ever again.

The Greater Good serving starts with me in *my* spiritual kitchen, cooking up meals of what I am the absolute best at. Any serving of Joy I wish to do begins with me leading by example, with me being at my best.

I have since discovered some cool ways to halt the normal, every-day tension between serving my Self and serving others.

Once we have some space between our Selves and a fear, an obligation, or some guilt that is weighing on us, we can clear them out of our life if we take the time to just think about them.

When I journal, there are three antidotes for clearing unnecessary FOG that I've used as tools to help me do this—gratitude, drilling down my whys, and self-compassion.

1. The antidote to fear is gratitude.

This is when I write down any fear I have that is lingering and place that fear in a "box" in the center of a blank (on both sides) page in my journal. Then I find all the pieces within that fear that I can be grateful about and surround that box with them.

I excavate all the lessons I've learned within that fear, all the things

I know now that I didn't know before.

I shift my focus to all the information, technology, and help available to me that I can be grateful for, to systematically, piece by peace, help me transcend a fear.

I search until I find at least one thing I'm grateful for from that fear.

I might be grateful for learning that sometimes I need patience. I might be grateful for realizing I am strong. I might be grateful for learning self-love. I might be grateful for knowing how to be in tune with my body. I might be grateful for discovering a new self-care tool.

I might be grateful for the learning and tools that trained me to become more confident in my ability to eradicate new fears.

The more trained experiences I have with placing gratitude around a fear, the more I grow my intimate knowing of Joy in my life that helps me dissipate my fears.

Over time I have become fear-less…and it has become easier to place fears in a box and get rid of them.

When I am able to extract the tools and what I've learned from my fear, and place some gratitude around it, the process shrinks the fear and empowers me to transcend it with a newfound sense of power… from centering on what tools are positive for me and knowing what I didn't know before.

If I do this on a separate piece of paper, when I've finished with a fear, I can "throw it away" when I'm done and keep all the discovered gratitude for future use by cutting the words describing the fear out of the page.

I've done this process a zillion times, and I have far fewer fears in general because I have strong lessons of what I've learned from previous fears that can be transferred to any new fears to dissolve them.

2. The antidote to obligation is drilling down my whys.

As I said earlier, when I deal with the obligations that I have in my life, I start with the reason *why* I must do something.

Then I look for the reason behind that reason. And then I look for the reason behind *that* reason. And so on, until I get to a reason that resonates very strongly with me.

I don't stop until I get to the reason why I will do it or won't do it.

The reason that resonates deeply with me is the absolute strongest reason why I must do X—whatever that is. Here is where I find out what I choose to do or not do, with no obligation.

In addition to saying yea or nay to an obligation, I can simply change the context of my obligation.

For instance, when I'm invited to go to dinner with somebody, but I'm feeling obligated, I ask, "Why do you feel like you have to go to dinner?"

"Well, because they invited me, and I said yes."

That's not a good enough reason.

So, I keep digging deeper with my reason: "Well…I'm feeling like I *should* go, because I haven't seen them in a year, and I really should see them."

Still not a good enough reason.

I have to keep going: "All right, I haven't seen them in a year. I feel like I'm obligated to see them, but I don't want to do dinner. I'd rather go out to a movie."

Now I've changed the context of the visit.

Now I don't feel obligated to go to dinner, but I actually want to see them. Because going to a movie with them is actually something I want to do with them.

I realized I was sick of going out to dinner, and I wanted to go do something different and still see them.

I can choose my obligations with my awareness of how I want to assign my time and energy to each activity. Each one of my obligations is a separate task, and each one can be chosen through the "yea, nay, or just not today" filter.

If I have emails I need to respond to, phone calls I've got to return, errands I have to do, I ask myself, "Do you really need to do each one of them today? Do you really need to do each one of them this summer, this week, this hour," etc.?

Once I've made my decision, released my Self from the obligation I've chosen to do or not do, or just not do today…once I have a good enough reason to either do it, not do it, or postpone doing it *for now*… the feeling of obligation dissolves simply into activities I do or don't do or do at a later date.

When we are not aware of what resonates with us, we can come up with reasons to fulfill excessive obligations; we can get all the way to the end of our last breath doing these things at the expense of what we truly value.

I make sure my reasons are good enough reasons *for me*. A good enough reason for me requires me to have the power to live out my values.

It can't be just a good enough reason for the other person, or the group, or whoever, and I'm simply "obligated" to do it. It's got to be a good enough reason for *me* to do whatever it is I feel I must do.

At some point, my reason might change or evolve. My reason can change in an hour, by the end of this chapter, by the end of this year. It all depends on where I'm at and what's going on in my life.

That's okay. As long as I find a reason that resonates with me as to why my reason changed, I discover I am constantly enjoying my tasks. I will release my Self from each one of those obligations, until I find my Self…having *none*.

3. The antidote to guilt is self-compassion.

I can clear a lot of spiritual debris from my heart if I go through the things from my life that I carry guilt about and release my Self from them.

I do this by recalling any guilt that I am still carrying. I try to remember something that is tethered to me from my past that I feel guilty about. I imagine I am back at the age when the experience happened, and once again I'm that person.

I might be 13 years old, talking back to my parents, and I still feel guilty about that. I might be in my twenties, making a mistake that I haven't forgiven my Self for. I might be in last week's meeting, beating my Self up for my faux pas, etc.

I dissolve the guilt around that event. As I carry that moment, that event, that experience...I carry that "guilty" person right beside me, within me. I might be a little ashamed about it, or I might just have good old-fashioned generic guilt surrounding it.

Either way, I need to dump it. To do this, I practice a little copy and paste compassion.

For example, if I'm 13 years old, I think of a 13-year-old; or if I'm in my twenties, I think of a 20-something; or I think of a friend who is my age from last week, and I copy and paste that person onto me at the time that I'm remembering.

It can be anyone. I just want to find whoever, a relative, a neighbor, a TV character around the same age, and copy and paste them onto me in that experience.

Now I bring them *out* of that experience by sitting them down in my imaginary living room in my journal and telling them what they need to hear.

What am I saying to that person about their guilt? What do I need to teach them? What do they need to know that I know?

I sometimes start the conversation with some "it's okay" bathing; i.e., "It's okay, you didn't know." Or…"It's okay, it wasn't about you." Or…"It's okay, it wasn't your responsibility." Or…"It's okay, you did the right thing." Or …"It's okay that you took care of your Self."

The words *It's okay* coming from the Voice of compassion are very powerful words to hear with our heart and absorb into the bones of our knowing.

We want to shower each piece of us (that 13-year-old, that 20-something, that person from last week) with self-compassion to wash away the excessive guilt tethering us to the past, so that all the pieces of us can come into the present with us.

We need to speak to them. And say what they need to hear because we might be carrying their guilt with us, and they need our compassion.

We need to speak to them, if we're carrying their pain inside us from when they were age 13, or in their twenties, or from last week.

We need to speak to them, because they deserve to *know* they're loved, understood, and forgiven by *us*.

We're so quick to give that compassion to our family and friends. They show up in our living room, and we tell them exactly what they need to know to heal, but sometimes we find it so hard to do that for ourselves.

We must include our Selves in the compassion we so easily dole out to others. Self-compassion releases us to be present with those we love and gets rid of the guilt that tethers our souls to the past.

I have done this for all the guilt that I have carried. I have written in my journals what my younger Self must know about my experiences and rid my spirit of the guilt surrounding them.

Once in a great while, for some lingering traces of guilt, I do this copy and paste compassion process just to re-bathe myself in all the self-compassion I need, to free my Joy to be present completely.

Our Body Boundaries

To me, heaven on earth is real.

Because I am living a heavenly life on my quiet little spot of earth, and I have the time and energy to spend developing the ideas I have, to do the things I want, make the art I imagine, play with the people I love, with *time and energy to spare*.

I own a life steadily filling to overflowing with more Joy, less stress. Along with the heaven I now experience, I have been taught by the repetitive abundance flowing into my spiritual cup, that there's still more contentment on the way.

My cup runneth over…and over…and over. I am being taught… the well just *won't* run dry.

I find my Self evolving within *the freedom of my own power*, and I am blown away with gratitude for the gift of time and energy in which I can do this.

This gift that my newfound freedom has provided me has me experiencing ever-spiraling Joy, right here in my humble abode, in little ol'

West Gardiner, Maine, US of A. I now write and teach and paint and entrepreneur and play with the most peace I've ever had.

With this grateful, graced-filled, great fulfillment that I feel, I focus on connecting with my Greater Power System and always strive to emanate from—originate from—this greater connection, as I write and teach and paint and entrepreneur and play at my life.

When I listen to my intuitive Voice and discern directions with my GPS that guides me, I hone my "hunches." I explore solutions to problems or answers to questions that I then study the results of with those "tips," those "pushes," those "inklings." Positive results hone the right Voice; negative results confirm the wrong direction. Positive energy empowers me; negative energy obstructs me.

This continuous stream of "miracle" data informs my work as a mind-body-spirit and wellness, guided-journaling instructor. I find myself the recipient of some kind of never-ending cosmic donation of paradigms and visuals and language tools that endow me with all sorts of simple, helpful, transmutative, grounded insights…to grow my life and the lives of those who co-create with me.

Intuition can be so powerful when trained. All the intimate comfort I receive from blossoming my original ideas into pure Joy-filled satisfaction, fills me daily with fascination. The metamorphic linguistic beauty of guidance is delivered so personally to me, creating such intimacy with me. It's sort of like having the local florist show up daily on your doorstep with bouquets of flowers, all with cards signed, "With love, Joy."

Over and over, I recognize that I have been relentlessly sent the same message from my GPS into my journals that was revealed to my mother—you are loved, you are seen…and yes, you are worthy of Joy.

I say *relentlessly* because there were also a thousand times when I wrote in my journals about how I was all alone—how I felt profoundly excluded…resigned to a depressing belief that deep Joy was not in the cards for me like it was for others.

But in fact, upon reflection, lying right there in black and white… were the words from my GPS downloaded into my journals, flowing through me, infusing me, connecting me…*course-correcting me*, with guidance toward understanding my worth through the growing Joy in my life made evident within the records I kept.

It seems we spend our lives pursuing so many endeavors, chasing all kinds of dreams. All the while, we walk around with this fluctuating hope, and sometimes fragile belief, that a Greater Power System exists to help us. But I think what we'd really like is the steady *certainty* of it.

We can go about the practice of experiencing that consistent assistance for our Selves more frequently (like I do through guided journaling) by *intentionally* cultivating a deeper flow, within nature, prayer, meditation, music, art, language, science discoveries, math breakthroughs, sports challenges, transcendent events, shared rituals, spiritual places, good works, good people, good ideas, and so forth.

Access to a greater connection with our GPS is *everywhere*.

We can hone our intuition all day every day. We can find our own entry point into the flow of the river that pulls us in out of the disconnect, out of the stresses about the past and the future, and carries us completely inside the present moment down the river of Joy, in whatever way satisfies us the most.

We can find and form new flow habits within everything that brings us deep Joy. We can find and master a regular practice of engaging with whatever Joy flows *through* us, leaving our spirit washed with excitement, cleaned with satisfaction, and our lives thoroughly soaked in hope *verified*.

Hope becomes verified when imagined dreams come true and envisioned expectations get fulfilled, visualized plans get accomplished, and conceived ideas get birthed, raised, and matured into *satisfying* Joy. When hope becomes verified, there's a sense that you just ate a spiritual meal that was absolutely delicious.

Hope becomes verified when our "Maybe it's possible" is transcended with, "This desire, this dream, this *debt* is...*done.*"

I personally experience that thorough Joy when I reach the peak of pleasure with my art, or when the light within my students' eyes "turns on" during the courses I teach, and my hope in reaching satisfaction is *finished w*ithin me.

I also acquire thorough Joy with the connection I experience in regularly taking in Maine's many gorgeous sights, where hope in absorbing peace and beauty is finished within me. And with the reciprocity I receive from the amazing people committed to doing their jobs for me in my businesses, where hope in achieving mutual success is also finished within me.

All these are experiences in the spiritual river, flowing into the Greater Good ocean that truly raises my Joy, resuscitates any hope that feels like it's drowning, flips the upside-down scarcity in my life rightside up, replacing suffering with miraculous abundance. It has been a buoyant miraculous abundance that *replaced* my temporary reality of "Relentless stress is sinking me" with the permanent wonderment of "Nonstop flooding of Joy *keeps raising me.*"

Sometimes I find myself questioning the recurring miracle data, scratching my head, saying, "What the hell?"

But then the repetition of time with Joy rising in my life crescendos, and it hits me: "Oh, *wait*...this is *heaven* on earth!"

We may learn what Joy we desire in our lives by learning from times of stress what we *don't* want in our lives. But the absence of illness is not always the same as having health. Time with Joy is necessary to know what we *do* want in our lives.

Spiritual health requires that we exponentially, *consistently*, raise our spirit with Joy by actively experiencing transcendence in flow habits, from within our Selves and from within those we are in relationships with. We can progress our spiritual intelligence and mature our intuition even more by intentionally cultivating *more* Joy from consistent satisfaction achieved from time with Joy.

It behooves us to not just seek Greater Good help during times of stress, but to also train our Selves to develop a deeper relationship with our Greater Power System and evolve our Joy.

This happens when we *receive* abundance from our Greater Power System, and we *share* equitable abundance with our Greater Power System, which returns to us an even greater abundance of time with Joy, cementing the collective *knowing* in us that we are not alone.

You have a greater power that is *yours* to co-create a Greater Good with, if you choose. That same power also resides in every single other person on this planet, if *they* choose.

But our choice to co-create must be made in a reciprocal environment. It's a universal right, but it's not always universally exercised.

The intention behind the doors of our universal right to choose to co-create must exit the spiritual home with inherent knowing that we are included. Our efforts must originate with the Greater Good in mind…and that effort must include us fully.

Getting comfortable with how big our shares are in humanity's mutual fun requires training across time with Joy.

Training in mutual shares of intentional Joy enters our lives every day, nonstop. The dividends paid to us from within the Greater Good… the inclusive time with Joy…can comfort us thoroughly and persistently.

I grew up with the Father, Son, and Holy Spirit of Christian origin as a great source of comfort to me. With maturity, I discovered several other enriching paths as my sources of comfort. I put the origins of what I receive from them all under the same umbrella labeled: Spirit.

When I say *spirit*, I am referring to both our collective human spirits and our innate universal spirit, all of which guide our actions within our intuition, our Voice, our Joy, our *knowing*.

There's the human spirit part of someone's character that we experience, as in school spirit, team spirit, community spirit, national spirit. Or the broader aspect of spirit that we recognize, as in the spirit of law, the spirit of cooperation, the spirit of humanity, the spirit of celebration.

There's also what I call an "uppercase" Spirit, with a capital S—a sometimes unnamable, Joy-raising guidance system that humans use in many ways to guide their behavior and experience transcendence.

The sources of our guidance systems can be any faith structure, ethics system, Greater Good structure, set of guiding principles, transcendental systems, etc. But to co-create within the Greater Good, our guidance system should include us in the co-creation of more Joy, less stress.

The commonality for me in teaching more Joy, less stress, is that we all strive for experiences of transcendent Joy as we live, love, learn, and leave a legacy with as much satisfaction and fulfillment as we possibly can.

When I refer to a higher power as a GPS that guides us, it's like the GPS in our phone or in our vehicle. We choose a destination, and the directions come from a "satellite" view, a Greater Good perspective… the instructions we need get downloaded. The communication, like our intuition, our Voice, our Joy, our gut instinct, directs us.

And rather than just referring to this accessible power as a *higher* power, creating only a vertical relationship structure, or as a *wider* power…creating a horizontal relationship structure, I refer to this power as a Greater Power System that balances the two.

Our GPS has the goal of heightening the Greater Good, yes, but also of broadening the Greater Good. *Both* you and I get to heighten and broaden our Joy.

In my courses, I teach a simple perspective to guide the students toward hitting their self-care targets by heightening and broadening their Joy.

Instead of viewing yourself as a human body, housing your mind, your emotions, and your spirit, view yourself as made up of five bodies: physical, emotional, mental, social, and spiritual, with the spiritual body being independent, yet also flowing or "running" through all the other bodies.

For a visual, I draw four solid circles and place one of the "bodies" in each of them, with the spiritual body encircled in dashed lines. I then take dashed lines from the spiritual body and "run" them through all the other circles and back to the spiritual body, sewing all the bodies together.

The spiritual body is independent in its own circle, but it's not restricted to that circle. It is running through all our physical, emotional, mental, and social experiences, connecting all of us together, via our spirit...actually, more specifically, by the Joy in our spirit.

That Joy is experienced through the "invisible" intentions of people, the "unseen" aspects of the human character, the "hidden" inner workings of humanity, the "spirit" of you and me.

The solid boundaries encasing our physical, emotional, mental, and social selves remind us our body boundaries allow us to be independent humans. With the spiritual body flowing through all the bodies connecting all of us together, any unsolicited effort to make it past our body boundaries is also experienced and discerned within the spiritual body.

It behooves us to remember that the origins of the power to protect our body boundaries, the *knowing* of our *no*, comes from the Joy personally experienced and trained with our spirit, telling us: this feels good…that does not feel good; this sounds about right…that just doesn't sound right; this looks correct…that doesn't look correct; this tastes amazing…that tastes awful; this smells heavenly…God, that stinks.

These are all events experienced within our physical, emotional, mental, and social bodies, but also judged as positive or negative for us within our spiritual bodies.

If we are raised in empowering environments, we reach adulthood with Joy as our ultimate tool to see, smell, touch, taste, hear, and *sense*, to know the character of a person, the intention through their body language, the context of their acts.

We must have the training to discern how a negative or positive experience is affecting our body. And we must have *the power to decide* whether an experience is positive or negative for us.

We must also have the training to fully embrace evolving positive transformations that occur within the Greater Good.

What may be evolving in one body needs spirit to help the other bodies to also evolve; i.e., when we need to change our environment, our diet, our exercise, our feelings, our mind, our job, our Self, our community…we need our spirit, connected to our Greater Power System, to get our entire body on board.

When we have an experience that feels good in one body but doesn't feel good in another (i.e., mentally but not emotionally, or socially but not physically, etc.), we need to pay attention. Our spirit is our connector; it will tell us when our physical, emotional, mental, and social bodies are not all in agreement and provide direction with how to get the whole body…*whole.*

Our spirit is what connects all the information together, collecting all the good across our physical experiences, our emotional experiences, our mental experiences, our social experiences, to first lead us to a collective knowledge, to guide us in defending our collective boundary, then to help us develop a collective knowing.

For example, I learned some boundaries and then developed my knowing regarding my physical body with two experiences I had growing up.

The first was when I was 8. I had one of my close friends over to play and we ended up in the bathroom, sitting on the floor with our underwear off, looking at our body parts. My mother came in and was angry and broke up the exploratory party. She let me know in no uncertain terms that she felt that behavior was wrong and was not to be tolerated.

I felt her anger, and I connected it to my physical body. My physical body was wrong to look at, touch, and pay that kind of attention to, according to my 8-year-old mind.

It wasn't until I was an adult that I pried apart what was so wrong about it. As a child, I thought my physical exploration was wrong. As an adult, I learned that it was the complete opposite. It is a natural and necessary part of connecting my body to my spirit.

As an adult, I understood my mother's anger. I was with my 8-year-old friend, and she didn't want to cause trouble with the girl's family and be embarrassed—she was uncomfortable.

As an adult, I pried apart what were healthy and unhealthy body boundaries. As an adult, I reset all my boundaries to include my complete comfort with my physical body.

The second experience was when I was in high school. I had gone to a party before a dance, had too much to drink, and got a ride to the dance with one of my male classmates. In the parking lot, before I could get out of the car, out of the blue he put his hands down my pants, and I found myself fighting to get his hands off me.

Just as he did that, a female classmate was walking by and saw what was happening. She walked up to the car window, banged on the glass, and yelled, "Hey, Anne, the dance is already starting!"

The boy quickly let me go, and I jumped out of the car and ran into the school. (The girl that came to my rescue just so happened to be the same girl from the bathroom panty party.)

As a child, I quickly dismissed the event, putting it out of my mind and my body. Later, as an adult, I learned that I had been sexually assaulted. As an adult, at first I was ashamed of my naïveté as a teenager.

But also as an adult, I connected my body to my spirit by exercising self-compassion for that trusting nature I had in me as a child. As an adult, I reset all my boundaries to include safety protocols in drinking alcohol, while *retaining my trusting nature*, and I've since added appropriate boundaries that protect my body thoroughly.

As an adult, I have mastered, with my GPS's directions, my nos and my knows.

With so few instances of my boundaries being violated, I recognize the spiritual upbringing that laid the groundwork for me in learning all my body boundaries from time with Joy. I recognize time with joy connected my spiritual body to the rest of me, and the training in this connection originated with several remarkable Greater Power Systems—my local church community, my school, and my family.

My church community was quite charismatic. The role models I had provided me with the structure of my Greater Good relationship within a Greater Good system. My school was the source of so many great memories.

At every mass, I was embraced by many members with enthusiasm and respect. In every class, I was treated as smart and having something to contribute. At every event, I was transformed by the power of spirit flowing from the leaders into all our activities.

I learned to love and feel loved. I learned to seek, express, and *expect* Joy.

I learned to volunteer. I learned to care. I learned to teach what I learned. I learned from a lot of good examples how to *become* a good example…of being and doing good.

My family was also (and still is) a very empowering force in my life growing up. These role models I had provided me with the knowing of my roots, the health of my childhood soil, the bounty of my family nutrients…that made up the tree of my life.

My parents were the bridge connecting me to my church, my school, and all the rest of my family. Patriarch and Matriarch, side by side, leading by example with, "Listen to your spirit, Anne. Go ahead and play in peace…you've earned it, Anne."

They were very active in my life. Through their values and their joy, I learned what my nos and my knows were. I felt so able…so *capable* with them.

My mother was a master at helping me bring an abstract, "unknow-able," gray-bearded, ethereal God down to earth and into an intimate relationship with a connective tissue system that formed the structure of my guiding principles and bound me to my intuitive Voice, within the Greater Good.

My mother taught me to reach *deeply* into my senses, to feel Spirit alive and accessible inside and around me…and to feel this sharable power flowing through me so I would experience Joy as *real*, not abstract.

My father was a master at making me feel loved, smart, and beau-tiful—by the way he held me, by the way he treated me.

On a multitude of trips, I used to sit between him and my mother in the truck, while Dad gave me a map and said I was in charge of the directions to get us where we were going. Talk about empowering the

GPS in me! (And I'm aging myself with the era of no car seats for kids.)

When I was a little girl, his CB trucker handle for me was Pretty Princess, and as I was growing up, he called me that all the time. I loved going for rides in his big semi truck, which had my name along with my mother's nickname on the front of it.

He took me out of school to play hooky (arguing with my mother that I was doing well enough in school to take a day off) to go tour sawmills for ideas to develop his mill. (I love that he found me interesting enough to take me along for rides with him, just so he could talk with me.)

He took me out of school (making sure I had all my schoolwork assignments ahead of time) so we could go up to camp in northern Maine, to take spontaneous vacations, to travel and see beautiful sights together.

He loved to take me fishing. He once bought my favorite chocolate-covered donuts and woke me up at 4 a.m. to go fishing with him and my brother...only to come home laughing from the terror of getting chased off the pond by an angry mama moose protecting her baby. He built a trout pond behind our house, where I fished in the summer and skated in the winter.

I took ice skating lessons both before and after school and trained for competitions. Both of my parents would go skating up at the rink with me on the weekends. During the week, Dad brought me to the rink for practice before school, and Mom brought me to the rink after school.

The rest of my family, my school, my church...all provided me with lessons in time with Joy just as my parents did.

I just felt so cared for and cared by and cared about by my parents and my family, school, and church community. (Talk about drip-feeding the physical, emotional, mental, social bodies with the safety and *freedom* to know Joy.)

Our boundaries take effort to develop, make no mistake, and we sure can sleep well in our homes at night when we know *what* they are, *where* they are, and *when* they need to be established.

And in reaching adulthood, the accumulation of the presence of Joy through all the seemingly small experiences of my life…being trained in what a whole spirit feels like inside of me…helped me immensely to not feel so starved of heaven on earth during times of hell.

The collective power of all those Joyful and mystical experiences infused in me the knowing, the *reality*…that a deep and abiding shared Joy includes *me*.

It is this Joy that I also share, that I pay forward to bring my *community* body together, because I believe in my ability to heal, hold, honor, help, and heighten Joy in those open to receiving it.

Most of us can agree on the experiences we share of awe and transcendence felt throughout our lives.

We *know* the essence of when we have a universal spiritual experience, even if we can barely articulate what it is. There are a zillion words and images that attempt to describe what we are experiencing, to define when we are in the presence of that unnamable *quality*.

Joy is in both the river we ride on and in the entire ocean we bob around in. Joy is in both the tree we hug and in the forest we traipse through. Joy is in both the air we breathe and in the gravity we all dance in. Joy is in both the heat we warm our bodies in and in the sun we all see with. Joy is in both the planet we share and in the universe we evolve in.

It may take a lifetime to get to know Joy intimately and totally through time. The best we can do is connect to its power, become whole, and share the experience of that wholeness so others can enjoy its miracles too.

A human being, being human, is a complex, nuanced, multifaceted *wonder*.

We are frail, yet we are the most powerful creatures on earth. We are small in the universe, yet we loom large in our power over this planet. We make mistakes, yet we have the most power to correct them. We have excessively fragile egos, yet we repeatedly transcend our fears to shrink them. We are a whole species, yet we can routinely celebrate one single, *passionate* person. We have holes in our perfection, yet we manage to love perfectly.

I find us to be a miraculous species. As we grow up, we can mature our spiritual capacity. As we raise our Selves up, we can evolve our spiritual tenacity. And I *know* as our entire body thrives, we can grow our spiritual audacity.

Coming All the Way Home

Self-care *habits* are crucial to maintaining the spiritual home.

It isn't enough to put the peace-puzzle of our lives together once, we also need to have the capacity, tenacity, and audacity to *keep* the pieces of our Selves intact over the course of our lives. To maintain our wholeness, to continuously feel total and complete and not let any part of us go missing.

We need to upkeep our physical, emotional, mental, and social homes so we can enjoy a spiritual home that provides for, nurtures, and protects the Joy in our lives.

We need our self-care habits established to keep all the pieces of who we are intact, to stay at home in every way, to live our fullest lives everywhere we go, with everyone we meet, with everything we do, every day.

The home as I speak of it here is your entire body *filled* with *you*, filled with your spirit, your Joy, your complete satisfaction. Home is no one else but you, owning your body. Home is in your total freedom with being *fully* alive. Home is every bit of you *present* in your body.

Home is you sitting fully in the space you take up. Home is you moving through life filled to the rafters with Joy. Home is you being completely at peace with your life.

The home is *all* the pieces of you *connected.*

The home is your physical, emotional, mental, and social bodies woven together with your spiritual body, fusing you into one whole human being, being fully human with *Joy.*

A key piece of keeping you whole, keeping all of you home, is learning the distinction between unnecessary stress vs. full Joy and the effect they have on your self-care habits.

Sometimes to maintain our Joy, we can institute *good* stress in our lives. A good stress is a stress that brings us *satisfaction*, not pain. It strengthens us, not hurts us. It helps us, not strains us. It mends us, not breaks us. It's stress, but not really.

It's a chosen and empowering demand upon our body that includes gentle stretches, appropriate challenges, mastered skills, and balanced needs. Meeting the demands of any of these can make our Joy *fuller.*

Good stress is temporary, short-term, with an endpoint that stops when the "enough" threshold is reached. It's stress that makes us *feel good*, not bad.

Good stress also inspires and motivates and focuses our time and energy, and it positively, proactively progresses us with the satiation received from our satisfaction.

Like the stretch of a deep tissue massage, the challenge of a workout, the skills learned on a new job, the emotional tools we mastered to be a leader, our needs balanced within a relationship. All these examples are temporary stresses with finish lines that bring us home to our best Selves.

In contrast, unnecessary stress goes on and on. It can be a good stress, but at some point, it crosses over into "too much" territory. Or it's just an unnecessary stress from the beginning and it doesn't let up.

Unnecessary stress has no endpoint, no cap. It just keeps going and doesn't feel good.

Unnecessary stress can become an abusive pattern that chips away at the Joy in our lives, wearing down the fullness of us—our home—unless we put a stop to it, or we depart from it.

These patterns are stresses that cause us pain. These patterns are stresses of excessive wear and tear on our bodies. These patterns are stresses of struggles that become repetitive. These patterns are stresses of emotional labor taking its toll. These patterns are stresses of relationships that dismiss, discard, or discourage *how* we need to stay home.

These patterns are stresses that can bend or break your self-care habits, that can negatively affect the size and shape of the pieces of you, making them not fit into your peace-puzzle anymore.

These patterns are stresses that make you leave your best life, that make you miss who you are, that make you crave who you want to be, that make you throw away the Joy that you value.

Keeping our Joy intact with demands on our bodies that *fit* us, requires us to have fully developed intuition. When we encounter unnecessary stress, we have to have fully developed intuition to provide boundaries, to nurture, and to protect our physical, emotional, mental, and social self-care habits.

The limitations of our human bodies must be cared about, the nuances of our needs must be cared for. We don't want to live a life where we reside only partway home.

When we are pushed out of our own homes of Joy, when we are pushed beyond our capacity to maintain our own wholeness, when we are pushed to endure missing pieces of our own Selves, then we miss all that brings *us* Joy, and our self-care habits can suffer.

We need *our* self-care habits in order to be fully at home with our spirit.

Missing pieces of our Joy, missing the full Joy of our lives is not to be endured, and if it is, we must make changes in our lives to get our Selves the rest of the way home.

There is unnecessary stress that gets us to leave our inner home—where we are centered in our values, at peace with who we are, enjoying the life we have…less and less and less, until we are rendered home-less.

We need to eradicate or depart from this stress and come back home.

There is unnecessary stress that may cause us to leave what we value behind, to abandon progress we've made, to say goodbye to Joy we've accumulated, because a stressful person wants to move themselves, inch by inch, fully into each room of the empty life we've left behind.

We need to say goodbye to *them* and come back home.

They may entice us to stay home-less physically, emotionally, mentally, socially. They may lure us away from the home of our values, the home of our self-care, the home of our Joy.

They may coerce us to stay home-less physically because they want us to leave our home to go tend to them, to the "relationship."

They may charm us to stay home-less emotionally because they want us to leave our home to keep *their* mood upbeat and calm.

They may persuade us to stay home-less mentally because they want us to leave our home to invest our intellect mostly in *their* dreams.

They may appeal to us to stay home-less socially because they want us to leave our home to make *them* the center of our attention.

They may repeatedly discard, dismiss, and discourage what brings us Joy, and render us home-less.

These can be stresses that sneak up on us.

We become home-less from the stress of being forced to live everywhere but where our spirit calls us.

We become home-less from reminders of what we cannot do or have or be.

We become home-less from the lack of assistance in helping us to get *our* dreams finished. We become home-less from being forced to ignore *our* needs and relegate meeting those needs to a "tomorrow" that never comes.

We become home-less from our desires always just *barely* satiated. We become home-less from our deepest missing Joy numbed with substitutes.

We become home-less from our unmet needs due to a relentless list of "more important" needs that must be met first. We become home-less from our Joy missing, because too much energy is required to retrieve it from under the pile of someone else's needy debris.

We become home-less from our needs "met" over and over with just words and never any action. We become home-less from our needs missing because of plans, plans, and more plans…that don't include us.

We become home-less when the smallest of our lost desires go missing for months and years and decades. We become home-less from our depression because a stressed person placed our missing Joy within our view…only for us to *hope.*

Discerning unnecessary stress requires time and energy to notice whether it has become a pattern of discarding, dismissing, and discouraging our Joy.

An unnecessarily stressful person reduces the full space we occupy in our lives by moving us as far away from our home as often as possible to make room for their insatiable needs.

In extreme circumstances, if we attempt to clear the unnecessary stress to return home to our Joy, and it causes a stressed person to get excessively angry because we implemented intuitive integrity-maintained boundaries, their negative energy can feel like a bomb dropping on the spirit.

They can create a wasteland of toxicity that is cancerous to remain in. They can pollute our spiritual home so much that we have no choice but to get out of the relationship. The relational "home" has become uninhabitable.

In addition to making sure I don't develop a habit of spending less and less time home, I have learned it is important to live, love, learn, and leave a legacy in a home with Joy fully present. I have developed self-care habits through activities I experience that make my spirit rise.

Making my bed up daily with pretty pillows in colors and patterns and textures that I love makes my Joy soar. Spending time daily learning something new that interests me excites me. Enjoying frequent travel in my home state lifts my mood tremendously. Teaching weekly line dancing in my community stokes me.

All these are self-care habits that sustain deep Joy in me.

In our everyday lives, whenever our deepest values get fully realized by staying authentic with our Selves, we satisfy our soul. We feed our spirit, bring peace to our whole body from the sense of coming all the way home with our deepest Joy.

To help us do this, we can live alongside positive spiritual SWAT team partners.

Part of choosing positive spiritual SWAT team partners is seeking those who do not throw away our instincts, who do not disregard our intuition, who do not dismiss our gut feelings, who do not dump our Voice, and who do not trash our Joy.

Coming spiritually home requires us to have a solid foundation to build our homes on, along with a solid framework of SWAT team mentors to teach us what a beautifully maintained home with self-care habits looks like.

Our spiritual home must be provided for, nurtured, and protected. The cohesion of us and our Joy and our Greater Power System becomes the good bones our self-care habits are built upon.

We must maintain the health of the bones of our knowing—our intuition—so no part of our body suffers needlessly. We need our entire body fully connected to our spirit, to feel completely at home with our Joy. The connected spirit is the glue that holds us all together.

When we're discerning what self-care habits are right for us, part of our job is to tear out the negative that creates havoc with our lives, keep what we love, and open our Selves to new Joy that gets delivered to us from within the Greater Good neighborhood.

Our GPS will do just the opposite of a stressful person. It will lead us *away* from patterns of discarding, dismissing, and discouraging our Joy.

Our GPS will seek to help us retrieve every missing part of us, so we will never experience home-lessness. Our GPS will repeatedly lead us home to Joy in perpetuity, evolving us fully while we live, love, learn, and leave a legacy in the safety of our GPS's shelter.

Our GPS will teach us that we do not have to leave our spirit behind to keep our home, to maintain our self-care. Or that we do not have to ever leave home behind—our self-care—to keep our spirit.

Our GPS evolves us through our learning, gathering, and down-loading Joy perpetually. To finish what we start, to then learn more Joy and finish that Joy, and then learn even *more* Joy and then finish *that* Joy.

And on and on we go, building a full life with no unnecessary stress, with no home-lessness.

You can share your passions, your skills, your ideas, your successes with your partners, your families, your coworkers, your community at large. Your constant Joy will be our teacher, your best habits will be our models. This is the yummy stuff we need to institute self-care habits for our Selves that speak to *our* spirit.

People *know* Joy when they see it. People *know* when you're spiritually home because they feel your integrity emanating from your body, your character, your actions, your *habits*.

They know when you consistently lead from a place of innate generosity that envelops them with Joy also. They know when you're home because they also can come spiritually home when they're in your steady presence.

There are humans starving on the planet in need of people who are home. They are in need of a steady diet of synchronistic experiences, transcendent experiences of Joy, community, comfort, and protection in their daily lives. You can show leadership in feeding their needs by sharing your best self-care habits with them.

We each can leave an old home-less experience behind; we can take the experience and remember it through the lens of self-compassion and then recognize the growth of our Voice from it.

We can put it in a different light and release it entirely to the past, and then come home.

We can enter into homes with experiences that lift our soul and recreate any part of them for our Selves and adapt them into self-care habits for us.

We can fit all the pieces of the Joy habits we need into our self-care and then come home. Come all the way home.

If you can believe in the magic of your life
and let the possibilities float to you,
as you gain confidence in the wisdom of your soul
and let your inner Voice teach you,
you can be present within each moment
and let your life unfold before you.

Follow the Path
of Joy's Persistence

(This chapter is a journey through my own journals.
My hope is that as I strive to find and learn from my Voice,
I might also enlighten and inspire the possibilities within you.)

I feel so small today.

It's such a big world…and I feel so small in it.

I feel like I am one…in a sea of many. One solitary soul who dares to dream, but who cannot fathom the universe parting the seas…just for me.

I sit here perched on the ledge of my accumulated knowledge and talents, on the brink of a new beginning. I sit gazing out at the future of unlimited possibilities wondering, *Just where will I fit in?*

I wish I could climb the trees high enough so that I could see the forest around me. I wish I could get a clearer view of how my life might eventually turn out.

I have searched and researched what my destiny is to be in life, and all I have are bits and pieces. And every time I think I have enough pieces to complete the puzzle, there seems to be more to the picture.

Is this universal? Spending our lives learning and discovering ourselves, honoring our talents and gifts, achieving our goals and dreams, thinking, *There's* my purpose and legacy…only to find ourselves simply growing beyond them into new ones.

Am I the only one who seems to live life repeatedly peeling off layers of myself—slowly revealing who I truly am?

Am I the only one perpetually graduating?

Today, there's a new path calling out to me, and I want so badly for it to be the right one. But I don't know if it's meant to be. I don't know if I have what it takes to create the life I dream of.

It's so hard to embrace a new path; it's so hard to let go of all that is easy and comfortable. It's such a gamble to put my Self out there, to risk stumbling and failing for everyone to see.

I think I resist showing my cards too early in the game because I feel like I'm still figuring out who I am. Every day, I am learning something new about myself, and when I think it's so new I should hold it in and protect it, I hold it in because I'm not sure about it. I don't want to display an aspect of who I *think* I might be. What would be the point if I wake up tomorrow and find out…nope, *this* isn't who I am?

I would only confuse people.

(*You mean yourself, don't you?*)

Yeah, well…I feel like I have the whole world in front of me and I can't seem to find my way. Something is affecting my Compass; there are so many voices, with so many possibilities, trying to steer me in the "right" direction, I'm getting disoriented. I can't seem to find the missing *peace.*

Am I headed in the wrong direction? Should I turn back and go a different way? Did I take a wrong turn and get lost? And am I really lost, or am I just afraid?

I think I am more afraid.

And as I look out at the different paths, as far as I can tell, there's no hint as to which direction I should go. The trails ahead of me seem to wander aimlessly.

I have been trying hard to blaze my own path in this world. I have been trying hard not to just blindly follow those who have gone before me, but I realize I am truly lost and afraid. And I think being afraid keeps getting me lost. I think being afraid is blinding me. Something tells me that even if I could find the path I think I'm supposed to be on, I'd still misplace the courage I would need to stay the course.

And if that's true, where exactly do I go from here?

I'm not sure, but I need to clear my head. I want to download onto my journal pages all my thoughts and feelings as they bubble up to the surface, see if I can clear away some of the fog that's obscuring my way today.

And while I'm there, I'd like to look back through my journey to see if I can get a better perspective of my life. I'd like to explore whether there is a common thread running through all the times I was the happiest and most fulfilled. I'd like to see if I can figure out when and where I felt the most clarity, the most at peace: What was I doing? How did I get there? (Never underestimate the wisdom of your own journey…)

Well…after reading and writing through my journals, I thought I was on the way to discovering a big aha moment of clarity that would reveal how the pieces of my life are supposed to come together. But in searching for some wisdom that might point me to the finish line, I have been led to the starting gate instead.

It seems that whenever I have to make a pivotal decision in my life, whenever I reach the edge of all that is familiar and stand at the gateway of the unknown, instead of trying to see so far down the path, I find my bearings when I simply focus on *one* step…And that is the step I take to connect with my spirit first.

I have discovered that whenever I take this simple contemplative step, whenever I pause long enough to stop, to become aware and heed my soul's Voice and become *present* with myself, it marks the *beginning* of the *end*…the end of my disorientation, my anxiety.

I realize this simple step has become the crucial foundation for all my clear and confident decisions. And if I want to figure out who I am and where I'm going now, I must first choose to practice contemplation.

Even though it takes a lot of energy to plant myself in my own presence, to quiet all the noises, to peel back layer upon layer of doubt and anxiety, experience has taught me it's worth the work to dig and dig until I finally reach the silence.

It's then that I can feel my soul's Joy, because, at last, it has been heard.

Experience has also taught me that practice doesn't make perfect— it just makes *peace*. My journals have reminded me how much I grow as I practice listening to my soul's wisdom. I can see the courage I gather, the trust I gain from embracing my own Voice, because I've learned that the enlightenment it provides *is really all I've ever had to go on.*

And I realize that, by trusting this Voice, I can choose to practice patience. I can grow my dreams beyond my fears and my anxieties and let the possibilities of my life float to me. One step at a time, I can explore the landscape, try something new, and learn what speaks to me, see what brings me closer to my wholeness. Then I can choose to stay with the experience until it teaches me all I need to know.

And then I can choose to practice surrender. Surrender to all those times when life made a choice *for* me, and I found myself someplace completely different from where I thought I'd be.

Whether I like it or not, experience is continually teaching me to trust—trust that I will be sent all the teachers and opportunities I desire, trust that the only thing I have control over is *this* moment... and my *Joy* in discovering it.

Hmm...I believe I have received a revelation.

It seems I have been equipped with a compass all along: *my Joy.*

It seems that whenever I pay attention during the times that my life feels at its fullest, when I pay attention in the times my heart sings its truest, in times when the peace within me is at its greatest, the guideposts I need are revealed in whatever it is I am doing in those moments.

I am realizing that my forest, my world, has become too dense with choices. But if I just pay attention to those times when I get *lost in the Joy* of what I am doing, if I pay attention to when time seems to float by, to when my smile is at its widest and my laughter is at its loudest, I will be guided right to where I belong. I will find my way out of the forest, and I won't *lose my Self* in the chaos of the world. I am realizing that the only way to filter out all the false hopes, instant gratification, and borrowed assumptions of what is supposed to make me happy, fulfilled, and peaceful—the only way out of the jungle—is to follow *my Joy.*

I just need to clear my mind and my heart to see where my Joy is leading me. I just need to pay attention to the signs *within* me.

Yet today, even as I grasp the power of my Joy, I realize I am still afraid of the unknown. To continuously let my Joy lead the way is really hard when I can't see what the outcome will be.

Sometimes my inclination is to pick what I perceive to be a sure thing, even if it doesn't speak to me. I find it easier to just arrive *some*where, *any*where, so I can just park it, so I can at least have the *illusion* of a sure footing.

There have been countless times when I didn't trust in the simplicity and *power* of my Joy, countless times when I did so much extra work to ensure I was headed in the right direction, trying to do the right thing...so much time wasted because I roamed the woods stalling, pacing back and forth along the ledge of the unknown, terrified I would make a mistake.

My greatest fear is that I will get nowhere with the one thing that will bring me my greatest Joy. I think if I do this *one thing*, if I jump into this *one* terrifying possibility, I might fall, I might fail. I might make a big mistake that will throw me too far off course, and I won't be able to make my way back. And then what?

Would I be forced to abandon all hope of ever reaching the sweetest, purest experience of Joy? Would I be able to survive the heartbreak of such a loss? Would I be able to find a new path as joyful as the one I feel like I'm chasing now?

As terrifying as it is to not know where all this will lead, at this very moment...a new realization is dawning. I am becoming conscious of the fact that I need not be afraid of living without my Joy...because *I can't shut out its beckoning whispers.*

Every day it calls out to me, and it doesn't stop ringing until I answer it.

Everywhere I go, it is present...in everything I do, it hovers...and everywhere I sit, it joins me.

Here I am, afraid that I will lose it, that it will somehow be snuffed out of my life by the winds of the unknown, and yet I've realized that as surely as I am breathing, *my Joy will not abandon me!*

The possibilities that Life brings to me will always be evolving, the trails will forever be twisting and turning, but the *compass* I use to explore them will always remain true. Even as I am eternally changing and growing, my Joy will be constantly on the move with me... guiding me.

Looking back through my life today has helped me to see the

countless paths that have led me to where I am. And I realize that a lot of the choices that have thrown me off course have been the ones made in *fear*.

But today, I think I am less afraid of whether my decisions will lead me in the right direction or not because I am learning: All that's standing between me and making my way to a clearing is a *choice*.

How well I choose just takes *practice*. And with enough practice, I will learn. And as I learn, I will grow, and as I grow, I will arrive at new places, with new possibilities and new opportunities.

And along the way…I will grow a stronger, more confident Voice to *choose* with.

Today, the trek through my journals has reminded me that, while there's also some guidance to be collected from those who have gone before me, as well as those who walk beside me, I can only use them as spectators cheering me on. Experience has taught me that pursuing what makes *others* happy is the quickest way to lose my Self.

I can be the most attentive student, but ultimately, I must sift through the answers *within* until I am left with the path that feels most real to *me*. And this makes me mindful of the fact that I will need extra courage if I am to go against the grain of other people's opinions.

So, can I see now what my life is going to be about?

Nope. I have spent years exploring my purpose. And still I ask, what is it?

I have no clue. But I do have some clues about peace and happiness and fulfillment.

My history has shown me that following the path of Joy's persistence is not always the path of least resistance.

Some of the most amazing places I have ended up have been the result of a hard, gratifying, satisfying climb up over the mountains of doubt, disbelief, and disapproval. There's something magical about that moment when I stop to rest and look at how far I've come, to see how brave I've been to follow in Joy's footsteps—

and the view is breathtaking.

Where I am right now is the sum of all my Joy-filled choices and experiences, and as I walk the seemingly random paths, the pieces of my life become arranged in some divine order that is beyond my understanding. And that's okay, because what I *do* understand is that *destiny is paving the way.*

I don't need to see: I can *trust* that my life will unfold beautifully.

I realize now…the lost connection between all the possibilities in my life…the last missing piece that will complete this magnificent puzzle…the only one *leaving breadcrumbs worthy of following…*
is *me.*

~

Author's note:

I wrote this journal as my daughter, Vanessa, was approaching her high school graduation.

As a child, she was a voracious learner. I raised her with a lot of free time to pursue her passions and interests, and from this, she uncovered many talents, skills, and gifts, and learned a lot about her Self.

As the end of her high school education was nearing, she was looking forward to college continuing to feed her hungry mind, as well as the opportunity to continue exploring more of who she might become.

But as we researched schools and degrees and classes, she realized she had to start making some hard choices. Where should she go? What should she study? How could she commit to *one* path when she wasn't sure which one was the "right" one? How could she compress all that she loved to do into just one degree? And how would that *one* degree translate out into the whole world and still encompass *all* of who she was at the time?

It was during that time that I was recognizing my own graduation of a sort. My son was also finishing high school in a few years, and I realized I was on the brink of a new beginning—returning to the work world full-time. As a result, all the possibilities were overwhelming me. Like Vanessa, I had felt ambivalent about my own future as I saw the empty nest rapidly approaching.

Through the years of being home with the kids, I had also explored my passions and interests, and I had a pretty good idea of the things that made me want to get out of bed in the morning. But I quickly discovered that it was quite a comprehensive list. I had a multitude of Joy that was calling to me, and as I was exploring my options in the workplace, I found myself struggling with having to choose. I realized that every single one of the questions Vanessa had about her future could have applied to me as well.

Where do I begin? Where will I fit in?

The problem was that each path I could have taken would seem to satisfy only one piece of me. Choosing only one felt narrow and *wrong*. I had accumulated skills, talents, and knowledge that had become a big part of who I was, and it was in the *sum* of these paths where I felt the greatest Joy in my life. I really felt compelled to find a path that encompassed as many of the pieces of me as possible.

But the real world of finances and responsibilities loomed, and until I could figure out a way to reconcile my heart's desires with the basic necessities of living, I had absolutely no way of knowing whether or not I could choose the life I really wanted.

Could I have my cake and eat it too? Was I dreaming an impossible dream? Was I being too greedy and naïve?

At the time, I truly didn't know.

All I knew was that every time I revisited planning for the future, I heard this persistent whispering Voice that just wouldn't let up.

So one day, to alleviate my stress, I decided to write in my journals and take an inventory of my life. I wanted to gather and understand the parts of me that made up who I was, and I wanted a better idea of how I had ended up there, with that nagging voice in my head and in my heart.

My journey led me all the way back to my childhood.

I remembered that when I was a little girl, I dreamed in color. Countless nights, I would fall asleep to lustrous, radiant, colorful scenes swirling around in my head. Sometimes, I would spend my days noticing all the nuances of colors and textures in *everything*. This was such a natural part of me, it wasn't until I was much older that I realized everything in my life was filtered through this lens.

And I also remembered that, as I grew older, I dreamed in words. I would wake up out of the blue with all these beautiful, meaningful words of inspiration and hope and *wisdom* pouring out of me. I would wake up with so much energy flowing through me, I could have gone out and run a marathon.

Sometimes I would write the thoughts down, staring at the words in amazement, my senses flooding with sheer Joy. I would sit in the privacy of my bedroom and reread them for hours on end.

Other times, I would get scared. I was in awe of the power of those words coming through me, and I didn't understand how or why I got them. At the time, I didn't tell anyone; I didn't want anyone to know… the mystery of it all, the power in my Voice on the pages scared the hell out of me. And because I didn't have a clue what to do with them, I would just tear the pages up and throw them out.

I looked back on this and realized that, even as I ignored this part of me, the words were quite persistent whether I wanted them to be or not. I remembered that this kind of power was hard to contain. I couldn't tell you how many times, after I'd received some inspiration, someone would talk to me about their problems, or their life, or their dreams, and whatever words I had received would be exactly what would slip out of my mouth—and be exactly what they needed to hear.

But as I approached the end of high school, my life got busy. I became too busy to stop and marvel at any cool words of inspiration; it became easier to just ignore the words. And over time, they retreated into hiding.

But for some reason, a Joy that I *didn't* push away was my love for art. I thought my natural eye for color, design, and texture would translate well into hair and fashion. So, three weeks after graduation, I followed that Joy and went directly into hairdressing school.

I really loved it, and at the time, I thought I would be perfectly content to do it for a hundred years or so, and I didn't think I'd ever do anything else.

But after working for a while at various salons, I discovered that a missing Joy was to be my own boss. I'd grown up with my family in business and was familiar with the lifestyle, and I realized it was calling to me as well. Everyone I knew from school had gone on to college, and I thought I should do the same and get a business degree. So I signed up for classes…and I lasted two weeks.

If there was ever a time when my Voice came in loud and clear and I didn't ignore it, it was when I found myself reading the textbooks from cover to cover, hungry to learn more, and realizing I didn't have the patience to sit still in a classroom for the rest of it.

I had worked in a shoe store throughout hairdressing school, and my instinct guided me to talk my way into an assistant manager's position at a new store that was opening. It was here that I discovered how much I really enjoyed learning hands-on. I soaked up all that I could learn about business, and a few years after that, I opened my own salon.

For twenty years, I loved it. I was able to feed my artistic appetite, and, as a wonderful bonus, I gained a lot of life experience, learning from everyone who sat in my chair. It didn't take long for me to realize just how much all my clients and I had in common—how incredibly individual and alone we all seemed to feel, yet how alike and universal the problems were that we all faced.

During that time, I had two kids. And in my free time, it was second nature for me to pursue extensive knowledge of something simply because I wanted to learn it. I had a voracious appetite for any interest that caught my eye, and one day, after months of resisting a radical new idea, I was inspired to pass that passion on to my kids.

I had decided to homeschool my children. I gradually scaled back my work, expanded rental properties for income, and closed the salon to follow this newfound Joy.

I think homeschooling was as much for me as for my kids. I had an outlet for my insatiable need to learn, and I had these cool little kids to share my passion with. I spent all my free time blissfully learning right along with them…teaching them the way I myself was still learning—learning things simply for the Joy of it. And, as a bonus, I got to spend a great deal of downtime playing with more art.

Homeschooling was a major turning point in my life, and it wasn't a clear path by any means. In the beginning, I was a train wreck; I was neurotic about crossing my t's and dotting my i's, obsessing over whether my kids were "keeping up" with public school.

It took some courage to follow this particular path of Joy because, in the beginning, I was met with a lot of resistance, disbelief, and worry from family members. I didn't blame them. There were many times when I was home with my children and would slip out of my Joy coma and go, Oh My God! What am I doing? Have I lost my mind? What if I screw them up royally? What if all my passion for learning isn't catching?

What if I'm not enough?

It didn't matter. I was called to do it anyway. I calmed down after the first few years and just let my *children's* Joy lead me.

Homeschooling was hard work but intensely satisfying—joining endless field trips, visiting endless places, digging up endless resources, all to keep up with whatever their current passions were, as well as introducing new ones. Whenever they burned out on one subject and picked up something new to dive into, I was off in search of whatever I could find to stay ahead of them.

What fun.

At the onset of this idea of homeschooling, I went through a great deal of trouble *ignoring* it. But everywhere I turned, someone or something would present itself, directing me right back to it. I ignored this calling for a full year before I finally answered it. All I knew was that every time the idea of homeschooling presented itself to me, *it just felt right.*

Despite being terrified of the unknown future, I chose this path because it was persistent as hell. It's one of the most important things I ended up doing in my life with so much clarity and peace.

I finished their schooling. Both kids are happy, whole, educated, and, most importantly, passionate about following *their Joy.* It's one of the things I'm most proud of teaching them.

I hope my journey toward authenticity inspired my children, because I believe this is the most important thing I will ever teach them. Be who you are. Do what speaks to you.

I'm not talking about the impulsive voice that demands its shortsighted, selfish indulgences, but the recurring whisper that doesn't let up for decades, the Voice that keeps reappearing in your sleep, in your daydreams…and in your *Joy.*

My journals took me on quite a trip. They gave me the perspective

I needed to see that it took me forty years of following my Joy to end up back at the beginning.

Life led me here.

As a result of going back through the experiences that brought me Joy, I learned what parts of me I could discard and what parts of me I couldn't let go of.

I learned I am happiest when I'm self-employed; I am happiest when I do art in some form; I am happiest when I am growing and learning about life. I am happiest when I spend time with my family and friends; I am happiest when I am able to teach and inspire…and I am happiest when I follow my *Voice*.

And during the time of this journal, my Voice was telling me to *write*. I realized that those words of hope and inspiration had lain dormant in me for too long, and it was time to *purposefully* follow them.

At the same time, I was also feeling called to start selling some of the art I had been designing. So along with my daily journal writing, I started exploring and using simple words and phrases on the art that I was creating. My initial intention was to focus on simple affirmations, to offer a spotlight of inspiration that would be a daily reminder of the beauty and truth in all of us.

It didn't take long before those words weren't enough. I found I had *more* Joy in expanding the beauty and truth of those words with even more depth, conveying an even more profound meaning of my intention. I wanted to better convey the power of words we could really dose ourselves with, to amplify the power we felt so we could further inject it in others.

I found myself simply continuing to follow my Joy, surrendering to all those words that had set up camp inside of me so many years ago. As the Voice inside of me grew, the words also grew…into lines of poems and strands of thoughts. And then the lines began to gather together into clumps and form paragraphs and stanzas.

And the words kept coming—lyrical, beautiful, empowering words. Either alone or strung together, a few at a time or as long strands of hope and possibility...until one day, I had completed an entire chapter.

It was in this moment that I experienced the full force of my own beauty and truth...and found my greatest Joy.

Currently, I write books and teach guided journaling and paint art along with managing rental properties and a few other jobs. I've started multiple companies that encompass all the parts of me. For now, the pieces of my life feel connected to a bigger picture, a greater purpose.

I used to have some tough, desolate days when I asked myself, "Should I really be doing this? It takes a lot of my time and energy, and I have relationships I don't want to neglect. I don't want any regrets pursuing a self-proclaimed, solitary, unproven calling. I have expenses to concentrate on. I can't afford to bypass a real paying job on an artsy, touchy-feely, cockamamie idea."

And I can't tell you how many times I used to "quit."

I would get overwhelmed with fear, exhausted, and discouraged with all the effort and decide to throw in the towel. I'd go a few days or weeks, and at first I was relieved to be rid of it, but it wasn't long before the Voice started nagging me again. I would sit down to write in my journal, revisit my thoughts and feelings about my decision to quit. And after attentive contemplation, I inevitably revisited the pivotal question: Am I supposed to be doing this?

And every time, my Voice answered, "Yes."

I had to do it. I couldn't *not* do it. Time spent with and without it has taught me this.

And I do it *every day.*

These days the Joy dam has broken me open, and it carries me away in its power. I am powerless to stop all the words and designs that come to me now. Every time I try to restrain them, I feel miserable. Whenever I try to shut them off, I drown in my chaos and misery; I become lost and apathetic.

My desolate days taught me that, even though I built the practice of connecting to my Voice on a regular basis, I also needed to build the practice of *trusting and relying on* that Voice.

I believe if we persevere long enough at pursuing the basics of life, there will come a day when we walk through the door of higher needs and are asked to embrace a higher calling.

Yes, we all need to address the basics of how we will live. But once those basic needs are met, we will feel this pull toward something greater, we will find our spirit *wanting*…imploring us to take the next step.

And I have learned that taking this next step—discerning a higher calling—is a continuous process.

I was reminded of that when Vanessa approached her college graduation. Even though she picked a path that was a combination of what Life presented to her as a gift and what simply felt right to her at the time, the process of her first graduation was repeating itself.

She was once again anticipating her future, wondering what decisions to make next. Should she go on to grad school or should she go get a job? What school would she go to? What job would she go for?

Her Voice leaned toward working, but there was still anxiety in that decision. I could sense her apprehension and her uncertainty, her questioning: Just where do I belong? What if I waste a lot of time in the wrong place? What if I take a wrong path and it ends up nowhere?

In witnessing this process, I recalled similar fears in my own graduation, wondering…Am I truly following the right path? Will I be able to thrive in my own future?

At the time, that remained to be seen. I just took it one step at a time; I just chose to thrive on Joy.

And it paid off. As I said earlier, I am living in heaven on earth now, continuing to thrive on Joy.

My experiences with graduating have taught me that the journey to my destiny is traveled more en*joy*ably with Joy present. As I learn and gather the pieces of myself, I can embrace Joy each time I discover a moment that fits me, while step by step I work toward creating more of those joyful moments for myself.

Some of my experiences are now big pieces of who I am, and some are now little pieces. But just because they're little pieces doesn't mean they're not the exact fit needed to complete the overall picture. I've done things for a short while, when I didn't like 90% of the work, just so I could gain 10% of the skills or knowledge I needed to add an important piece to my life puzzle.

I find I can only withstand the effort when I have my Voice to sustain me. That's why I practice guided journaling. Tuning in regularly with my Voice keeps my patience long and my focus high as I gain experience...*trusting* Joy to lead the way.

I've learned there's a big difference between gaining experience and making mistakes. Mistakes happen when I hear my Voice loud and clear and I *ignore* it, while experience is simply the manifestation of practice.

Only practice will fine-tune the balance between my self-care habits and the world. When I'm feeling lost and overwhelmed and small in the vast world outside of me, I reduce my fear by tapping into my GPS. With practice, the spirit inside of me grows in power and my fear in the world outside of me shrinks.

That's the beauty of practicing guided journaling...it builds confidence in your Voice. And with enough confidence, you gain the faith and *conviction* you need to trust that you are on the right path…and to exercise the *courage* to follow it.

With practice, it becomes easier to see when I need to abandon a difficult path or buck up and follow it through to the other side. With practice, I can recognize the paths that have the potential to be molded and shaped to fit me better and which ones look like dead ends. With practice, I learn how each path adds to my experience, and I collect more information about what makes me tick—I learn more about who I am.

I try not to beat myself up when I don't get it right—when I take a wrong turn. I try not to have regrets that it took me a whole week, a month, a year to figure out I was on the wrong path. I'm gathering experience…I'm gathering pieces of the puzzle that will give me more of the picture. Those times when I stumble into the wrong place… are simply teaching me who I am *not*.

I realize that when I think I've gathered enough pieces to see the whole picture, a shift happens. Whenever I stop to absorb an achievement, or sit to admire an accomplishment, the view of my puzzle zooms out, and I see that, as big a part of my life as this achievement or accomplishment is, there's so much more to the picture. It's then that I find my Voice urging me on to bigger and better things.

I realize that whatever I do will be pieces of a puzzle so large, *I may never get to see the whole picture.* The scale of what I think is pretty complete will be reduced by all the possibilities that still lie ahead of me. Maybe the overall picture won't come into view until much later in life, when hindsight can give me a bigger perspective.

In the meantime, I am a woman, I am a mother, I am a daughter, sister, friend, colleague, teacher, artist, writer, entrepreneur, and who knows what else might present itself. I am all or parts of these—sometimes full-time, sometimes part-time, sometimes all of the time, and sometimes just a sliver of the time. Big or small, if I embrace *all the pieces* that are equally important in creating me, I will feel whole, complete.

I like being whole. I believe being a whole me is *greater* than the sum of the parts of me.

Figuring out who I am is an interesting and ongoing trip. I am old enough now to realize I will never reach my destination. "Arriving" has such a short-lived satisfaction. It's human nature to strive for something better, to seek out something even greater, to graduate with *peace*.

Each day, as I travel forward, I bring with me remnants from each of the paths I have taken—lessons I have learned, skills I have mastered, and confidence I have gained. I find I can do a lot of things well. But experience has taught me that knowledge and talent alone don't define my purpose. Without Joy, it's just a good time doing something I'm good at while it lasts.

With Joy, however, what I do transcends my life. I can lose myself in it and, at the very same time, find my *Self* in it. *With* Joy, I find that what I do fills me to overflowing and empties me at the same time. As peace and Joy enter and flow through me, fear and anxiety pour out of me. It's out with the *old* and in with the *new*.

It's a divine exchange of energy, hope, and possibility. And as each new threshold presents itself, I can embrace it. In every single moment, there is an opportunity to go from who I was, to who I am, to who I want to be. Step by step, I have been gradually preparing for this moment…*Joy* has led me here.

Young or old, we are all in the same class together. We might approach a new beginning, a graduation, ambivalent and afraid because we are about to change who we are…into who we might become. But some graduations are simply turning points to take what you've learned about yourself and grow in a new direction.

You will encounter many fellow classmates passing along the knowledge that they've accumulated. Embrace them. But take their perspective…*and filter it with your own Voice.*

You are the only one who will know when an experience has run its course, when you've learned *enough.* You are the only one who will know when it's time for something new.

Take time to practice, to grow your own Voice, to evolve the Joy in your life. Gather those pieces of your Joy that you can claim as *yours* and share your Self.

And as new paths present themselves to you, remember you are *worthy* of embracing each Joy that calls to you…*Joy* is our equal opportunity employer.

*If the journey through your day is leaving you
without completion,
And the passage of your life is finding you
without satisfaction,
Perhaps the wisest use of your time
is in need of attention.*

Daily Peace Rises
and Sets Within You
>—<

(Another journey through my journals…)

You know what I just realized?

The more my life gets stuffed with things I have to do, the more empty and lost I feel. Each day feels like a giant black hole, and every time I try to take something out, something *else* wants to jump in and fill it up.

Every day starts with my mind attacking my list of responsibilities and expectations. And every day ends with my heart yearning for something more—something more meaningful, more fulfilling. One day just blends into the next. I fall asleep still hungry for my dreams… and I wake up with my mind already filling up with the day's tasks.

And today I am so overwhelmed, I don't even know where to begin. There's so much that I *have* to do, and yet there's so much that I *want* to do. Today, I'd like to put an end to this daily grind. But first I really need to whittle down the have-to-dos before I can enjoy any want-to-dos.

How do I boil the responsibilities of my life down so they don't feel so impossible to accomplish?

(*You need a big pot.*)

How do I find the time alone without such pressure to *do*? How am I going to find the time to even *think* about creating more time for myself?

(*You need a bigger pot.*)

And how on earth do I find time to reduce all the outside stimulation so my inner thoughts and feelings and dreams can bubble up to the surface of my life?

(*Uh…I think you'll need a bigger stove.*)

Yeah, well, I've been writing a lot in my journal, complaining about how tired I am, how stressed I feel because I have so much to do. How many times do I have to write about how busy I am? Complain that there is no time for me?

I'd like to go through my journals and highlight every time I've complained, because I'm curious as to how far back my misery goes. Along the way, I hope to find a revelation so I can put an end to all this deprivation. But what I really need is a miracle.

(*You mean like another one of you?*)

Wouldn't *that* be sweet.

Well, I am not finding any revelations within the pages of my life, but I *am* finding plenty of repetition. I can't believe I've been saying the same thing over and over for *decades*. There's not enough time for me…if I could just have more time for me…I can't find any time for me… ad nauseum.

I can see that the daily list never ends. I can see that whenever I get tired and stop, the list continues to grow, and because I can't find any relief ahead, I just simply press on.

And my despair remains.

I realize I have become crowded out of my own days. It has been so much work to hold onto anything I want to do for myself because if I force myself to step away from what I have to do, I am seduced back into it thinking, There's still more to be done and I *have* to do it.

And if there's any energy left over for me, any willpower residue that might help me resist my need to finish, I still surrender to the guilt of "Wait until the day is over, *then* you can have your time. You can't just leave this *unfinished*."

Of course, there is never any time left over at the *end* of the day. The flaw in this thinking is the "wait until the day is *over*" part.

This leads me to wonder, Why am I only getting the leftovers? When do I get to feast at the banquet of my own life? And why does "have to" feel so necessary, so nonnegotiable? Why does "want to" feel so selfish, so greedy?

As I've been trying to organize my time ever more efficiently and plan my days ever more effectively because I want more time for me, I realize that it's not enough to just *want*—I can *look* at my days and see that I choose otherwise. I can see that I've organized them so I don't simply reach the end of my rope, but I also reach for the *other* end of it. Then I proceed to jump through hoops to get through everything that I plan to accomplish.

(*You need to let go.*)

Yeah, well, if my history is any indication, I don't do that very well. It's scary stuff, letting go. It's like pulling my own skin off.

Hmm…I can see that I have work to do.

So why don't I do *this* work? Why don't I choose differently *right now*?

I don't think choosing differently is the problem; I think it's giving myself the *power* to choose. Because it's so *hard* to choose. I need way more *courage* to choose.

It's nearly impossible to extricate myself from the demands on my life. Everything feels so important and necessary, and I don't have the guts to abandon any of it.

I always feel like I should finish in a certain amount of time, but of course there's only so much time. And when the list grows beyond the time I have, I am forced to choose. The problem is, it's so much easier to cut *myself* out of the day than to say no to anyone else.

I always seem to start out strong, thinking, I can do this; this can be done on top of everything else. The problem is, I underestimate how much time it takes and overestimate how much energy I have.

Yes, I feel industrious when I'm achieving and accomplishing; I feel like I'm getting somewhere.

But herein lies the problem: I'm not getting anywhere I *want* to go. Why is this?

I don't know…It's clear that I place great importance in the things I have to do…but why?

Because they show.

Because all my achievements and accomplishments are tangible evidence that I have been a productive and useful woman, that's why. I think I "stuff" my days because I'm so afraid of who I would *be* without all the results of my have-to-dos. I've established a precedent, an expectation of what I'm able to do, and to scale any of it back would raise my deepest fear—that if I don't get enough *done*, I will never *be* enough.

Hmmm…

I believe I have just received a revelation: I think my self-worth has become too attached to my achievements and my accomplishments.

If I let the pursuit of my have-to-dos continue unchecked, if I continue to expect my have-to-dos to *complete* me, I will be led further and further away from my *Self*.

It will be impossible to discover a whole other side of me if I never explore the potential of what I *want* to do. And waiting for what I *have to do* to come to an end so I can embrace what I *want to do* is wasting precious time—*my life.*

If I want to stop feeling half alive, I need to stop dividing my life into compartments, with the have-to-dos warring with the want-to-dos like the Hatfields and McCoys. Conducting my life with only one half of me engaged is…well…*stressful.*

I can't continue to live a half existence hoping the other half of me will show up at the end of the day to assist me in *completing* my life. And I don't need *two* of me to get everything done: There can only be *one* of me—one *whole* me.

If I'm going to truly be at peace with my life, I need to order my days so I don't end up feeling so hurried and dissatisfied. I need to give myself permission to establish my own tempo and lower the volume of my expectations. I need to relieve *Time* of my impossible demands.

I need to remember that Time is the space between *this* moment… and the *next.* Space—with enough room to *breathe.* The setting sun does not need to be my cue to hurry up and get it *all* done *today.* Maybe I can leave some things unfinished for tomorrow morning, or next week, or next month, or, God forbid…never.

And maybe I need to let go of my *fear* of letting go.

Maybe I need to accept that I can't contain or manipulate or direct or influence my world as much as I'd like to. Maybe I need to sit here and remember all the times that I've had the courage to hand over the keys and trust that Life would get me where I needed to go—and I ended up exactly where I was supposed to be.

It's been so seductive, this illusion of control. I have spent a lot of time trying to command my days, expended a lot of energy trying to get the upper hand. And with this heady power, I have simultaneously oppressed my deepest desires. Why?

Because I'm delusional, that's why!

Because I actually believed that if I could just chain and tether all the obstacles out of my way, clear a nice clean path for the possibilities of my life, everything would be just perfect—all the have-to-dos completed, polished, and displayed for all to see and then all the time in the world to dive into my want-to-dos.

It is clear to me now that I need to empower my want-to-dos to be at *least* as important as my have-to-dos; I need to move them *up* the list.

But it still requires an astronomical amount of courage to think that if I choose to invest time in myself, it will ever amount to anything. That if I place myself and what my heart wants up there with what is expected and required of me, I can justify it.

Justify...*that* strikes a nerve.

Why must I build a case to justify my basic need to attend to a rising passion or my simple desire to answer the call of a recurring dream? Why must I build a defense for the right to follow Joy or seek peace?

And why must I be "right" about the choices I make? *Why can't I simply choose to answer the call?* Why can't I simply choose to accept the *importance* of the soul work that needs to be done within *me*? And how can time spent feeling so whole and complete *not* be right?

This time tug-of-war will cease once I stop everything I am doing and first *own* the life that I have been given. And to do that, I must *choose*. I must choose to recognize the value in my *being*, not just in my *doing*.

But to choose my Self first is an ongoing battle. I can't just choose one day and expect every other day to follow suit. I have to choose *every* day. Every single day, I must be conscious of what I do and choose. Every single day, I have to work on myself to challenge the belief that what I have to do should take precedence over what I want to do, and therefore who I am meant to *be*. Every day, I need to pay attention to how far down the list I sink...*because that's telling me how little I value my life.*

If I want to put an end to this daily grind, I have to start at the beginning—with me. I have to put *me* on that list. I have to take *some* time to think and reflect and sift through my life in order to figure out *what* matters to me, in order to *do* what matters to me.

And if I am to be present while I accomplish *any*thing that matters to me, I have to stop placing my self-worth in the end *results*…in the parts I have *no control over*. I have to believe in my *current* worthiness and allow *purpose* to drive my actions.

Purpose vs. results can be hard to discern; it can be hard to tell the difference.

While results are the targets, purpose provides a *direction* for those results; it is my *aim* as I pull back on the bow. Results are the endpoint of whatever it is I'm trying to achieve, whereas purpose is the reason *why* I am trying to achieve it.

And from past experience, I know it is purpose that will add meaning and *order* to my daily life.

Being busy with my daily life isn't the same as being productive with meaningful activity. I don't necessarily need to be less busy; I just need to live a life doing what matters to me. And in order to do that, *what* to choose must include *why* I choose it.

I must ask *why* I want to do the things I want to do; asking *why* reveals their purpose.

If I connect to an important enough reason for *why* I must do the things I want to do, then I will believe I *need* to do them. This will give my want-to-dos the *power* to transform into have-to-dos.

And if I know what truly matters to me, I will find the courage I need to *protect my choices*; I will stand my ground. And once I have reordered what I have to do…then I will be free to focus on what I *can* do.

Now I have the courage I need…*now* I know what's on the other side of letting go—freedom. And *peace*.

Focusing on what I *can* do keeps me in the present. Doing what I *can* do is a relief valve for when I have *too much* to do. Doing what I *can* do is the antidote to those times when I'm obsessing over what I *can't* do. Doing what I *can* do is the compromise with my daily resistance against what I *don't want* to do. Doing what I *can* do is the remedy for my shame in failing to do what I think I *should* do.

I understand now…my daily peace begins and ends with the mindfulness to attend to my *whys*.

And *why* will I choose to do *this*? Because *I* am worth *my* time.

Why am I worth my time? Because I believe every single living creature was created with a purpose…and *I am **not** the exception to the rule.*

I understand now…my soul just wants my *undivided* attention. From sunup to sundown. It wants me to hear its divine directions. It wants both my heart and my mind joined in *Its* purpose. It wants me to choose *It* first, last, and in every moment between. I just have to pay attention, and surrender to my Soul's wisdom, which knows exactly *what* I need to do, *why* I need to do it, and *how* I need to do it. It wants me to trust in *Its* perfection and accept that everything will finish according to *Its* plan.

It may not be *my* plan, but it will all be as it should be. The journey of each day is simply to enjoy the ride. It's really all *I* have control over anyway.

~

Author's note:

This journal came to light years ago when I was in the thick of raising young kids, volunteering, working, and trying to start a business. I was managing my daily to-do list as best I could. But one day I woke up and realized I was really stuck.

Up to that point, I had made a lot of strides with streamlining my to-do list, adopting all kinds of effective strategies to organize my tasks—prioritizing, simplifying, and consolidating my life. I had made great progress, but I was still, at my core, profoundly unhappy, and I realized I wasn't getting any *lasting* results from all my hard work. I was continuously stressed out from my daily life, and it was starting to affect my health.

I felt that I was clearly missing something, and I decided it was time to try something different. I thought maybe a professional perspective would shed some light on the peace that seemed to elude me, so I went to see a therapist.

My therapist was a warm professional—easy to talk to, patient, insightful with her guidance. I explained to her that my goal was to reduce the amount of overall stress I was feeling from all the responsibilities I had in my life, and that I wanted to have a fresh perspective on what could be adjusted within my typical day.

At each visit, we discussed what had happened since the previous visit, sorted out my thoughts and feelings about various events that had cropped up, made plans for course corrections, and put the stress surrounding them to bed. Most of the solutions were pretty benign—small stuff that I could quickly use to make adjustments.

Initially, I began to feel better about my life, but it wasn't long before the effort stalled. On my way home from one of the meetings, I realized I was still not truly happy. I still had two big issues I had yet to address: how to get more time to write and how to find more time to work out. Lately, I couldn't seem to find *any* time for either.

I went to the next meeting and brought this up. I explained how I could not find the time to sit and write or go out for a walk because my daily to-do list felt so pervasive and big. I explained that these were things that I *really* wanted to do, but I simply could not get any peace or freedom to do them until I got my to-do list under control. I wanted so badly to incorporate writing and working out in my daily schedule, but for the life of me, I could not succeed in making it happen…my crazy schedule seemed to trump my attempts every time.

I explained that whenever I managed to squeeze in time to work out or write, I would think about what I *had* to do, and I would either keep pushing off what I wanted to do further and further into the day until I ran out of time, or I would fight to stick with the writing and the walking, and then end up cutting them short because I felt there was an imaginary foot tapping impatiently, imploring me to hurry up and finish.

It was apparent that even when I found the time, I couldn't write or work out in *peace*—all the things I had to do felt like they were just sitting there, *waiting* for me to do them. It was making me feel hopeless that I would ever be able to get around to doing the things I really wanted to do.

After I spoke at length about how big a problem this was for me, my therapist paused and looked straight at me and said, "Reverse your schedule."

Not sure I had heard her correctly, I responded with, "Excuse me?"

She repeated, "Just reverse your schedule. Place the things that are the *most* important to you first in your day, *then* do all the other things you have to do on your list."

After a moment of processing this, I gave her a look of incredulity and said, "But I have *responsibilities*; I can't just *ignore* them. There are things that have to get done, and if I push them later into the day, I may not get them done in time. And I *have* to do them."

She reaffirmed her position. "I understand you run the risk of not completing some things. But you have some flexibility in your schedule…set aside the time to write and walk first thing every morning, and then prioritize what you have to do after. Whatever doesn't get done, just roll it into the next day. Yes, we live in a society that normally doesn't operate this way, but that doesn't mean *you* have to."

I sat there in silence, trying to absorb what she had just said. And then I blurted out, "*Are you nuts?*"

I couldn't even begin to entertain the idea of doing what I wanted to do *first*. I just couldn't see it happening. I felt I would be *endangering* the have-to-dos if I tried to first accommodate my want-to-dos. I had so much stuff I *had* to do…*every* day. How could I risk putting them off and having them pile up, or not get them done at all because I took some time first to do stuff I *wanted* to do? That would only stress me out *more*.

I felt that she didn't understand me…that I was the wrong person to give that advice to. I would have to rearrange so much of my life, it would be impossible. I felt that I had so many balls in the air, if I tried to make a major change like this, all the balls would land on my head and then where would I be…worse off than before. This piece of advice sounded so incredibly *indulgent* and absurd to me, I immediately dismissed it.

"No," I politely explained, "that might work for the average person, but it just isn't possible for me—with work and all the family, house, school, businesses, chores, errands, and tasks I'm responsible for, it can't be done. As it is now, I collect all the different pieces of my life onto a master list, prioritize it, and pick off parts of it every day. I spend each day whittling it down, and there's no room for a major overhaul. It's taken me a long time to figure out how to manage the schedule I have now."

She paused and then responded, "Next time you come, bring me this master list; I want to see it."

So I showed up at the following visit, sat in my chair, got caught up on events since the last visit, and then the discussion turned to my master to-do list. I pulled out several pages of notebook sheets, written

THE INTUITION MANUAL: BOOK 1

on both the front and the back, and handed them to her.

She looked at me and then at the sheets, flipped each one of them over, scanned them, looked back at me…and burst out laughing.

When she regained her composure, she shifted in her seat, started to speak, took another look at the list, and burst out laughing again. This time, she got to laughing so hard, she was rolling around in her chair, slapping her knee, completely unable to speak.

This went on for several minutes. Her laughter eventually became infectious, and I started to laugh with her. But I was also sitting there in honest confusion, thinking, Just what in the hell is so *funny*?

Finally, she took a deep breath and gathered herself long enough to say, "No wonder you're so unhappy—this list is *years* long. I'd be depressed, too, if I was trying to get all of this done. It would take a lifetime to get through this list. You really need to let some of these things go."

Her reaction to the volume of my have-to-dos woke me up to the absurdity of trying to *complete* the entire list. I had put *everything* on those pages that I felt needed to get done. From painting the deck at the rental property to weeding the garden in the backyard, to planning one of my kids' birthday parties, to booking the family camping trip, to washing the windows on my house and getting my hair cut and visiting my mom and making important phone calls and running errands and completing projects, and on and on. All of it was important to me and all of it *needed* to get done, as far as I was concerned.

Hmm…was it possible that I was being *unrealistic*?

So then I asked specifically, "How do I fix this? What do I do with everything on that list? It all *needs* to get done. And as much as I cross stuff off, more stuff gets added to it, so it *never* gets smaller."

She chuckled and said, "For just a little while, stop working on that entire list. Just looking at it is overwhelming. Break off a chunk of the master list into a *small* list; prioritize that chunk according to what's important to you, and then focus on doing *one* thing at a time. And don't think about anything else in that moment. Get up each morning and do *one* thing. Once you've done that, then look at the mini list and do the *next* thing, and so on. When your little list is done, go back to the big list and pull more from it, and then do it again."

I liked this idea. This sounded a *lot* less overwhelming to me. So I went home and that day made mini lists, and started working only from those.

It didn't take long to notice there were certain things on the master list that really needed my immediate attention that day, and with the time I had left over, the rest of the list could get picked away at.

Over time, I realized I never got to some items on the big list because they either became obsolete, got worked on by someone else, or I just indefinitely ignored them and outgrew my desire to get them done. But not looking at the whole thing every day certainly succeeded in reducing my sense of being overwhelmed.

Surprisingly, after a while, this master list got whittled down to one page. Then, as I continued to let go of more and more, lo and behold, my entire master list fit onto *one* sticky note! It felt much better to stop looking so far ahead and stressing myself out with the enormity of a lifetime of things I thought I should be doing.

I felt much happier, and I stopped my visits with the therapist.

After some time had passed and I had been working on my sticky lists for a while, I woke up one morning and realized my unhappiness was creeping back in. I realized I still had not resolved the problem of not writing and working out more.

This was revealed to me when I went to throw away a few of the sticky notes and saw on every single one that *everything* had been crossed off *except* for the writing and working out that I *most* wanted to do!

At this point I became depressed. I began to think, What is the *matter* with me? Why can't I simply do these two things for myself? Why can't I find the time to do at least *one*? I had all this success with simplifying my life and yet I've gotten nowhere with making these two things happen.

I became angry, thinking, This is ridiculous. And I became determined to do something about it, right then and there.

I placed one of the sticky notes with the two uncrossed items up on my kitchen cabinet right in front of my face where I would see it every day, and I *refused* to make another to-do list. I was going to look at that sticky note every single day until I did something about it.

I did it for *one* day.

The *next* day, I completely succumbed to the pressure of my responsibilities. I went right back to chiseling away at my have-to-dos and putting off my want-to-dos until, of course…I had no time left to do them.

Weeks went by with me staring down that damn sticky note, until one morning the conversation with my therapist and her advice came back to me: "Reverse the schedule. Put the things you want to do so badly at the *beginning* of your day."

I had grown so angry, I immediately sat down at my kitchen table, slammed my journal down and started to write…I was going to process this radical idea—to put what I wanted to do *before* what I had to do. After a few minutes, I paused from my writing…I got the sudden urge to get up and start flipping through some old journals.

After perusing some really early ones, I found that I had been writing and venting years ago about the *same* thing I was venting about on this day—not enough time to do what I want; my time was eaten up by what I had to get done. *Nothing* had changed.

This really got me thinking…I *really* need to revisit my therapist's advice and feed my *spirit* first, not the to-do list.

At that moment, I decided to go on a journaling marathon. I instinctively felt that this day was the day I was going to get some kind of breakthrough because I had had success in the past with finding creative solutions to my problems through my journal writing. I was so fed up and desperate to find a *permanent* solution to my problem, I cleared my schedule for the entire day.

I then sat down to write in my journal…asking myself, "*Why* am I still resistant to writing and working out? *Why* is it so hard? Why can't I simply choose to do what I *want* to do? I *want* to work out more and I *want* to write more but I feel like I '*can't.*' *Why*?"

I continued venting: "And while I'm thinking of it, *why* am I so attached to something I clearly can't seem to get done? *Why* am I putting myself through all of this? *Why* not just let these two items go? *Why* not be satisfied with the amount of exercise I *do* get in and the amount of writing I *do* manage to write? *Why* can't I let these items go like a lot of the other things I was able to let go of on my list?"

Then it occurred to me: because they *matter* to me.

I continued:

> But clearly, they don't matter *enough*, or I wouldn't be sitting here agonizing over this. *Why* do they matter so much that I can't let them go, and *why* don't they matter enough that I can get them done?
>
> *Why* do I want to work out? I realize there is a part of me that feels I *should* work out. Apparently "should" is not a good enough reason, because clearly I'm not working out like I want to even if I feel I should be.
>
> So…what value is there in working out that I'd be willing to move my life around to make it a priority? I can't say "better health," "longer life," blah, blah, blah, because those reasons

don't *resonate* with me either. They *should*, but they don't.

I have to find out what *does* resonate with me.

Well, if I look at what happens when I *do* work out: I love the energy I get from a vigorous walk. I love to breathe in the fresh air and the connection I feel to nature when I walk outside. I love to listen to music, or to books that expand my mind and make time fly by on the longer walks. I love the conversations I have with my daughter when she joins me on the trail.

I also love the challenge of learning a new dance when I do line dancing, and I love how I forget that I'm working up a sweat as my body concentrates on the steps to the music. I love how flexible and relaxed my body feels when I do my stretches and how strong my limbs feel when I do my exercises. I love how light and energetic my whole being feels when I do any of this on a regular basis.

Looking down at what I had just written, I realized there were a lot of reasons that resonated with me; they were reasons that *motivated* me. Enough that it made me want to stop the inquiry and go work out right then and there.

Which is exactly what I did. I went for a beautiful walk on the rail trail in my neighborhood. When I got back home I felt *amazing*.

I sat down at my kitchen table, grabbed my journal and continued writing.

Today I'm not stopping this dig until *all* the bones are uncovered. I realize that just writing all those reasons why I wanted to work out put me in touch with my senses and the memory of how it makes me feel during and after a workout, and it motivated me to drop everything to go do it.

But what about my writing? *Why* do I want to write? *Why* can't I write?

I realize that lately the main focus of my writing has been

for my book. And as much as I love it, it hasn't been going well. I say I love it so much—that it's important to me—yet it isn't on my have-to-do list like the rest of my stuff. *Why?*

Clearly, I just haven't found an *important* enough reason that resonates with me.

So answer…why do I love it so much?

Well, as I write right now, I am realizing how much I *love* chewing on a profound problem. I *love* figuring out how to get the absolute most out of my life. I love the challenge of taking large, complex thoughts and distilling them down to their essence. I love the hunt for the perfect word that conveys what I feel about something. Writing in my journal is my favorite way to get a satisfying mental, emotional, and spiritual meal.

But what about writing for *The Intuition Manual*? I can still feel resistance to this. *Why* haven't I been able to write the book? Do the reasons that resonate for writing in my journals apply to writing for the book, as well? I can write in this journal right now with complete abandon and Joy, and they're both journal writing. What's the difference between the two?

Well…writing in my journal has no expectations attached to it. It's always been for the sole purpose of feeding my soul.

No expectations attached…*that* resonates.

I just had an epiphany!

While I have all the same motivation to write the book, the book is a little trickier. Not *all* my writing is driven by the simple need to connect with my Self; that's not why I write the book. I also write the book because I have something to say that I want to share…something that I believe might help people. That's what drives me to publish. It is a purpose that resonates deeply within me.

The problem is, once I've pulled my writing from my journals and collected them into book form for the book, I then attach expectations and a certain outcome to it. Like earning some money and having people read them and the hope of sales providing a living wage, and on and on. And of course there's the basic need for validation, to be *seen*. That's a tough one.

I can see that these expectations make it harder for me to write. I am paralyzing myself with my attachment to the end results. I feel the typical peer pressure to *show* something for all my hard work…that the effort has to be *worth* it. And I find if I don't get the results I expect, I can subconsciously give myself a D– in self-worth.

I realize that, if I want to get rid of the baggage attached to my book, I clearly need to detach a living wage from my glorious journal time…and *my self-worth from the results*. If I find I can't make a living wage from my book, I already have other ways to make the money I need to keep writing. I already have all kinds of ways to reduce the burden of financial success on my writing so I can protect the sacredness of this activity and the Joy it brings me just to put it out there.

And I need to remember…I have no control over any of the outcome of my work; I can only put it out there and do my best to let people know it exists. I have zero control over the end results.

Connecting to the *purpose* of my book, and not the results, allows me to focus on what I really want—to just write and put it out there and teach it. Remembering the original purpose of my writing for the book *frees* me; it motivates me to rearrange my life to make it a priority.

As I write this, I can feel *these* reasons resonating with me…giving me the courage I need to move things around in my life so I will actually write more.

As I finished this exploration in my journal, I realized that I now had the strength and the focus—and the *detachment* I needed—to set my schedule to include more writing.

I closed my journal with the courage to reorganize my priorities and the peace to begin my day.

Every day after that, I was able to begin my day with both my writing and working out, and for the first time in a long time, I was much happier and fulfilled.

Until one day I got hit with a Crazybusy wave.

An urgent task came up that required my full attention, and it ended up consuming the whole day. It completely crowded me out of that day and the next, and for some reason, the careful attention to my want-to-dos disappeared for two weeks before I woke up to the fact that *I* wasn't anywhere on my list anymore.

I went to bed that night thinking, How did I let this happen? How did I slip back into abandoning my want-to-dos so easily?

The very next day, I cleared my morning schedule and sat down to journal again. "I went two weeks before I realized I had not been doing the things that really matter to me. Why did I do that? How can I prevent this from happening again? What's going to trigger me to stop and realize what is happening before I get to the point where I'm completely depriving myself again?"

It occurred to me that I needed to make a plan, a reconnection ritual for how I was going to keep my whys close to me, to keep their purpose and passion *alive* in me. I needed to create triggers that would connect me back to *why* I am choosing to do what I'm doing.

So that got added to the top of my to-do list: Create reconnection triggers to reset my course when I veer off track.

As a result, I have since added some journaling prompts—one of my new connection rituals—into my journaling. They are questions that I ask myself to help me get unstuck and refocused again.

For example, I edit my have-to-dos with, "Why are you doing what you are doing right now?" I ask myself this question over and over to drill down into my whys, removing the layers until I find an *important* enough reason. And then I make sure it's an important enough reason to *me*.

This helps me buckle down and get the have-to-dos done, or let something go completely.

I also tackle my missing want-to-dos with, "What is it I 'can't' do?" Not what I *actually* can't do, but what I am perfectly capable of doing but am *telling* myself can't be done, and I am *pining* over it because I want to do it so badly. I find when I ask myself this question on a regular basis, it really homes in on vague feelings of unhappiness and dissatisfaction.

And then I ask, "*Why* can't I do it?" I explore what else is *more* important. "Where is it that I am attached to an outcome? Where am I under peer pressure? What is important to me based on *my* values and beliefs? Have I attached my self-worth to something that isn't important to *me*, and I'm eating up all my time resisting the truth of this?"

And one of my favorites: "So…what is it I *can* do? Am I thinking *small* enough? What small part can I break off and do right now?" This helps to reduce my sense of being overwhelmed, to reset my button and detach myself from the outcome. And it shifts my attention to what I can do *now*, not if…when…after.

Currently, a lot of my journaling has the goal of reconnecting, and as a result, it often helps me to get an aerial view of my life. Stepping outside of myself—writing as a spectator of my own life—helps me to expand my perspective and see the bigger picture.

When I am "down on the ground" and overwhelmed, it's usually because something is too big for me to process. By getting some distance, the view of what overwhelms me becomes smaller, and therefore a lot less intimidating. It helps me to tackle a big have-to-do. It helps me figure out how to take it apart and get it accomplished (like remodeling several homes I own or revamping my website).

While this is very effective, there have been times when my want-to-dos have gotten kicked out of my day because I've done just the opposite with an expanded view —I've collected a group of *small* have-to-dos and grouped them together as a bigger whole, thinking it will streamline my time and effort…which a lot of times it does (like when grouping errands in the same town on one day or tackling chores in one big chunk).

But sometimes, while I realize any one task is not typically more important than a workout or a writing session, when there's a lot of different types of tasks to complete and they start to pile up, my stress level rises…I get overwhelmed by the sheer volume (like when I have to wear my mother hat for one task, then my business hat for another task, then my fundraiser hat for yet another task).

I respond by trying to group them all together as one big task that I think will get checked off quicker if I "set everything aside temporarily, just until I can get them done." Of course, when I treat them as one, it's *big*. The stress then becomes all-consuming because this "one" task is going to take me a long time to check off as "complete."

At this point, I slip into "hurry-up" mode. And for me, when I arrive at hurry-up mode, *this* trumps the daily things I want to do every time. Hurry-up mode devours my want-to-dos…*especially* my writing and working out.

This is when I have to get off the train, reverse my tactic, and think *small*. This is when I tear the big assemblage back down into bite-sized pieces and pick off one prioritized have-to-do at a time, while purposefully adding my want-to-dos back into my life again.

Now that I've been doing this for a while, I have discovered—*a want will quickly run out of fuel without purpose constantly driving it*. I have learned that being aware of my whys is going to be a lifetime challenge requiring daily attention in practice. I must *continuously* add purpose;

I must feed myself with a steady diet of reasons that resonate with me if I want to live my daily life doing what's important to me. I have to stay in touch with why I do what I do, hence the power of "why?"

I have since developed some flexibility with placing my want-to-dos first in my daily schedule. I have found that sometimes it works better for me *not* to try to do them first in the morning. A lot of times, I am entrepreneuring in the mornings now, and that's also a want-to-do for me. I've moved my other want-to-dos to a later point in the day. And that's okay. They are all still a priority to me, and they still get done. Prioritizing them in my heart and in my mind goes a long way toward ensuring they get prioritized into my schedule, even if they are not first on the list. I can mix them in with my other tasks and most of the time not have them get lost in the shuffle.

The most important thing I've learned is that reconnecting to my whys is not a "once and done." *This* task is *never* crossed off the list. Paying attention is the most important task I have to do every day. *Everything else* follows this. This is why I strive to make guided journaling take precedence over every other task I accomplish. I will often get up earlier to spend a few minutes with my journal just to be sure I stay in touch with the rest of my life.

I have also learned that I must intentionally choose to *slow down…* because I have discovered it's the *quickest* way to get really clear about the things I want to do, so the list doesn't keep me "doing" indefinitely. Reducing the speed of my life helps me to keep culling my life so I stay on course with what's really important to me.

And recognizing abundance—practicing gratitude…recognizing that I am *enough*—is part of the process of culling my whys. Practicing gratitude helps relieve me of the unbelievable stress of feeling I have to *become* all the time. As I take time to recognize what I already have, it parks me in the *present* and takes the neediness and desperation out of my wants…and lets me *be*. It helps me get off the "I want" treadmill and returns me to the "I have" mindset so I can give myself permission to rest for a while.

This is part of the daily stress of modern life. The desire for belonging, or not wanting to be left behind, can unconsciously drive our actions. We *have* to edit our lives. We have to do away with the distractions and the attachments and the peer pressure so we can make choices to do things because *we* want to do them—so that they bring *us* fulfillment—not because it's what everyone else is doing or thinks *we* should be doing.

We have to practice keeping the to-do list focused…not *crowded* with things that *other* people value. We have to be careful that we don't fill up our lives with things we *perceive* as important, when the to-do list makes us too busy and we get lost in the have-to-dos and the *think-we-want-to-dos* and the should-dos. We have to remember that what we would give everything up for may take saying a *lot* of nos. Our nos need courage…courage that can only come from the whys that *resonate*.

I have also learned that the balance between simplifying my life and not living in boredom is tricky. In our culture, we have the tyranny of choice and unlimited ways to upgrade our boredom and the pursuit of perfection. (Like when I dream about creating all these shiny new HGTV rooms, when what I really need to do is go through my house and simply *clean* it.)

Staying aware used to be a constant challenge for me.

There was one time, I woke up thinking I should go fold the laundry so I could be "free" to write. I managed to sit down with my pen and journal, but I picked up my phone instead to check for messages, and then I scrolled down some social media, and then I got up from the table and started to putter around the kitchen.

I was procrastinating. I was resistant to unhooking myself from tasks I hadn't realized I had attached my self-worth to. I was feeling that my journal writing was unworthy because I had forgotten the purpose of why I was writing to begin with.

Then I forced myself to stop and open up my journals, and I started to revisit my whys to get back on track.

On another day, I woke up without a lot on my mind, but I knew I was feeling unhappy, so I took the extra time to journal to clear my head. I discovered that actually, I did have a lot on my mind. I went two days without working out, and at the time I thought I was okay with it. Friday, I was simply too tired, and the day before I was too tired, and I used what little energy I had to clean the house.

But through my excavation, I discovered I hadn't been waking up refreshed. I had been pushing myself to stay awake at night because I hadn't been home to "nest" much. I didn't want to go to bed at a decent hour because I didn't want the next day to come because it was filled with a lot of nothing I particularly looked forward to. Then I noticed I was spending more money on "stuff" because I was too busy to pay close attention to what I was spending on. And I was eating junk because I hadn't made the time to make healthy meals. And the house was getting cluttered because I wasn't home long enough to stay on top of it. The projects were starting to pile up, and the laundry was falling behind. There was no time for my creative needs. All of which was raising my stress level.

Upon further writing, I remembered that within three days I'd had three different showers, a wedding, and company visiting, and all this had kicked off the whole downhill slide. I was doing a lot of running around, and I wasn't walking. Because I was *running...from task to task*.

Clearly, I got knocked over by the Crazybusy wave. I lost my way.

And the practice of connecting to the whys of what I had to do had been lost in the undertow.

I have learned since to practice paying attention.

Those days taught me that while our daily peace rises and sets within us, so too does our stress. The stress from too much activity and the volume of mindless "doing" and the sky-high expectations of our lives originate in the daily choices that we make. While we may allow the stress to rise within us, we also have the power within us…to set it *down*.

We live in an era of a million distractions and "urgent" tasks, but it's *our* job to strip it all away and pay attention to what's important to us. We may want the sun to shine all night to get it all "finished" but *at what cost*? And to what end? If it's not meaningful to us, then why the hell are we killing ourselves doing it?

It is inevitable that, every once in a while, we will get knocked over by the Crazybusy wave. Periods of change in our lives, or disruptions in our routine, while a rhythmic part of life, often catch us off guard and send us scurrying. But if we resist the ebb and flow of life and the challenges it brings us, we get caught up in it and our "urgent emergency mode" button gets stuck on.

Taking time out to ride a period of change doesn't mean drowning in its waves. It means getting out of the rough seas, climbing up onto the beach, and turning around to sit and look at it from a distance for a bit. It means catching your breath, getting some perspective, and soaking up a little sun to reenergize yourself. Navigating a Crazybusy wave well…for any length of time…means you need to step out of it periodically in order to go the distance.

It means recognizing that there is a time to *do* and a time to *be*, a time to work and a time to rest. But what kind of work? Purposeful, *meaningful* work. What kind of rest? Present, *mindful* rest. Even in the midst of a Crazybusy wave...*especially* in the midst of a Crazybusy wave.

There are all kinds of ways to shorten the length of time spent in a Crazybusy wave—to plan ahead and create reconnection rituals that will help you get recentered when it hits.

It could be a morning ritual like yoga, or meditation, or drinking your favorite coffee with your partner while indulging in the morning sunrise. It could be a repetitive reminder in your phone to reconnect, or journaling your whys, or reading uplifting quotes on your bathroom mirror. It could be sneaking away to the nearest vista and watching the sunset, or it could be hiking your butt up a small mountain to sit and breathe in the panorama.

It could be reading and rereading this book. It could be sharing this message and your intention to stay connected and to *slow down* with a friend. You could take turns keeping each other on a "purposeful" track. You could enlist the people you love to sit with you on whatever your "beach" is. *Just make sure it brings some meaning and Joy to your life.*

Whatever the method, create little triggers that help you to redirect your attention with mindfulness, to stop and think about who you are and what you are doing—and *why* you are doing it. After a while, the self-care habits formed by using these little triggers will be noticeably consistent and your want-to-dos won't get washed away by a Crazybusy wave. You will be quicker to respond and reestablish your equilibrium.

I understand that these days everyone is busy. A lot of people are pretty consumed with their own busyness. But in the wise words of my therapist, *you* don't have to be.

Just stop *doing* once in a while. Aim to make *being* a daily ritual of pleasure.

I think a lot of people in our society are ready to get *off* the speeding train, or else we risk arriving at the end of our lives exhausted, regretful, and depressed at how much of it was missed...or wasted.

Someone needs to set the pace for those around them to achieve a more meaningful, peaceful life—why can't it be you?

If you are surrounded by the "hurry up and do it now" team and you are waiting for them to slow down…will your life pass you by, with you being exhausted trying to keep up? And to what end?

If you get off, it might feel like you're getting "left behind." It might feel like something is "wrong" with you. It might feel like you are lazy, or selfish, or greedy, or unambitious, or just plain nuts. But a life with some time spent *being* will bring you more peace…it will be a life spent fulfilled, satisfied.

Being is *not* lazy. Being is *not* unproductive. Being is *not* wasting time. Being may look like nothing is getting accomplished, but being is just the opposite.

Being is stopping to catch your breath. Being is grasping the bigger picture. Being is filling up the tank with gratitude and "enough." Being is exploring and imagining the vast landscape of possibilities. Being is holding tight to the practice of *not* wasting your time…*or your life.*

Just because it looks like you are not doing anything on the outside, it doesn't mean you are not thinking and sorting and prioritizing and simplifying and deciding on the inside. You are cleaning out and organizing your internal closet where you store all of your plans, your intentions, your dreams, your generosity, and your commitments…to your Self and to those around you.

Guided Journaling

To hone and polish our self-care habits so we can experience the consistent peace of *being* within our Selves and within our community and not just do do do, we need to develop our *knowing*.

With guided journaling, or increasing our spiritual IQ, I believe there is a difference between information and knowledge and understanding and knowing.

In guided journaling, information is intelligence accumulated into one place, or, in the case of spiritual information—into one whole body.

For me, knowledge is the next step up from that information.

In guided journaling, knowledge is information made intimate for us within our personal experiences. It's when we have clear views of the data collected, and we are thoroughly familiar with that data. And in the case of spiritual knowledge—it's when we have personal possession of that information, from that data informing our entire body.

I believe information needs to be guided to where it becomes knowledge, which then must be evolved to where we *understand*.

In guided journaling, understanding is when we've discerned, interpreted, and expressed that knowledge and our learning is finished, or, in the case of our spiritual understanding—is when our physical, emotional, mental, and social bodies mutually agree with the collected knowledge.

But understanding then must evolve to *knowing.*

In guided journaling, to know is to experience repetitive Joy, from the results of intentionally exercising greater application of the capacities of what we understand, of what we've finished. And in the case of spiritual knowing—it's to evolve greater repetitive Joy that grows our power to *exemplify* further completion of our spirit within the Greater Power System.

When we get to a place of understanding, and then partner it with our consistent experiences of Joy shared within the Greater Power System, we arrive at a place of knowing transcendence intimately, thoroughly, and *permanently.*

We arrive at a place where the strength in our Voice is rock-solid, and the release from our Joy flows from us like a river. Where our *being* is fully present in everything we do.

When we pair our understanding with our GPS, when our understanding is intuited, then gut-checked, and our GPS verified…then we *know* we are being guided with Joy, both in our journals and across our whole lives … creating the intuition manual we use to cultivate more Joy while weeding out unnecessary stress within the Greater Good garden.

Our world has a vast amount of information for us, and all the spiritual members of our SWAT team within our Greater Power System are very knowledgeable and committed to helping us sift through it.

It is important that we seek this greater guidance to navigate all the human information entering our lives every day to hone and polish our intuitive power and enjoy the miraculous results our intuition manual delivers. We need to not make decisions without the miracle data included.

When we team up together, our stronger-together connection drives us to arrive at our more-Joy, less-stress destinations, knowing we are not alone.

When we are connected to our GPS, it leads and directs us step by step, inch by inch…developing our understanding to the greatest heights of knowing.

When we are practicing guided journaling, deep "see" exploration of our journals can be a very efficient method of progressing every area of our lives.

Guided journaling is so effective in getting us more Joy and less stress because it's a keystone habit.

Keystone habits are habits that are known to increase other positive habits and greatly improve the quality and productivity of our lives— i.e., eating breakfast, making our bed, getting seven to eight hours of sleep every night, exercising regularly, etc.

When I journal, I date each entry. I don't waste precious time grammar-policing my writing. And I keep it in a private place, so I hold nothing back on the page.

Guided journaling is not a Facebook post or a community bulletin board; it's not a diary where I list the day's events.

It's a *guided* journal, where I write, speak, and learn from my experiences, by exploring meaning and significance with the Joy in my spirit and by growing the knowing of my possibilities from promises that are kept, achievements that are made, and potential that is fulfilled, that evolves my Joy.

The personal experiences I have with more Joy, less stress then becomes my personalized, actualized, Greater Good-verified, intuition manual guiding me, constantly evolving my life with more Joy, less stress.

I don't exit the journal stuck in any spiraled negativity; I want to end each entry with a positive outlook and feeling to take action with in my life.

I want to exit the journal with a proactive mindset and a sense that completion is now knocking on my door.

I want to open the door to that sexy, attractive partner named Completion knocking at the door, that's my positive proactive progressive date, offering me more Joy, less stress than I believe is even possible.

I want to answer the call to venture out from my journals and truly *live*.

I endeavor to journal enough to keep my self-care habits in tip-top shape.

I often journal on anything to just get my thoughts out in front of me. I've been journaling on notepads, the back of receipts, index cards, the back of junk mail envelopes, anything I could get my hands on when I didn't have my journal handy. I rewrote them or inserted the pages into my journals later.

If we harvest our journals often, we get spectacular results with more Joy, less stress. Harvesting our journals is simply going back through them to extract knowledge from our entries.

It helps to have our journals indexed in some way. I have most of mine indexed by the year. We can leave the first few pages empty of each new journal or add a sticky note to the inside cover to index/label major events in each journal when we finish them. This allows for easier finding and reviewing and harvesting patterns across major life events or seasons of our lives.

Our words reveal patterns, both positive and negative, and it pays to notice them. I use my intuition to guide me to which journals or which pages to peruse for more insight into my Self.

We can notice the sticky thoughts—the words that we got stuck on and found our Selves reading half a page down, realizing we don't remember anything we just read.

That stickiness is our cue to back up and explore that entry.

We can pull out our current journal and write about that sticky thought and see if it leads us to new insights. We can highlight the journals, tab them, explore the patterns of them. We can keep an empty page or sheet with us as we peruse through those pages to make notes and answer these questions:

Does the pattern strengthen our spirit or weaken our connection to our spirit?

What's catching our attention? What stands out? What's sticky? What resonates?

Did what we wrote then still ring true today? Ask our Selves why or why not?

What is missing from the pages we are reading?

Are we missing Joy? Do we need more patience? Do we need to set more boundaries? Are we dying to manifest something?

Is there time and energy with peace, to satiate the hunger to repair, maintain, and improve our self-care?

Across our entries, are we repeatedly avoiding something? Are we resisting something that is persisting? Is there something bothering us, nipping at our heels, and we can't quite put our finger on it?

Are we trapped in the throes of someone's doubt training? Doubt training is when someone's thick FOG (fear, obligation, guilt) mixed with the deepest of indifference, attaches to our spirit and leads us to doubt our Voice.

Do we have things in our days that don't speak to us?

Are we in the throes of gratitude abuse? Gratitude abuse is when someone blankets us in a FOG so we "learn to want" the things that they've "provided" us, that *they* value, not us.

Who can we reach out to for spiritual SWAT team partners that will help us obtain enough Joy that we value?

Are we able to progress the Joy in our life, to get us the experiences that grow our knowing enough, for us to gain more Joy with sharing?

Do we need to carve out time to write until some clues surface as to what to ask our Greater Power System for help with?

Is our Voice trying to chase us down to help us manifest something, and we are running in fear of it?

Along with tapping into our Greater Power System, we can sit down and face that fear with our journal…release and process that fear, so it doesn't have so much power over us.

We can really get a lot of harvesting done when we take some time to notice repetition in our sentences.

Are the patterns of our setbacks abusive, or just challenging? Are the patterns of our "challenges" relentless, or temporary?

Is the information we're processing proactive, or delusional? Is the eddy we're in internal, or situational? Is the conflict we're clearing within the Self, or relational?

We can pick a problem, or a nagging thought, or a pattern of behavior we desire to explore and pick a time frame to reread them and decide whether we want to harvest them.

If it's a positive pattern, we can experience the Joy from rereading them as they lead us to self-affirmations. (For instance, I've harvested entire lists of my successes to keep on hand for when I've had times I felt like I was failing.)

Do we see any connections to broader themes and patterns, but don't have time right then and there to dig deep into them? We can write notes of what is jumping out at us and save them to digest later, when we come back to put the pieces together.

We can tape an envelope into our journal and put the pages in it, for us to go back into later and get updates on our perspectives.

If we never reread our journals, we will still experience guided journaling just through the act of writing; the process of guided journaling is first achieved in the downloading of our thoughts, even if we never go back and reread them. Getting the thoughts out of the invisible realm and down into the visible realm in front of us is the first step in downloading.

Harnessing our free-floating thoughts down onto paper unscrambles our self-care priorities. In the courses I teach, we emerge from class with a clear sense of direction, a newfound sense of energy. Our downloaded thoughts paved the way for us to take action.

During the retreats I host, we emerge from our journals to continue guided journaling verbally with each other. Sharing our downloaded thoughts expands the possibilities for us.

Guided journaling is not a substitute for a SWAT team, but it is a fantastic partner in forming self-care blueprints in which to formulate plans with the SWAT teams in our lives.

We can emerge repeatedly from our journals guided with which action to take with our lives. We might call a therapist to get an issue processed, schedule a meeting with a manager to present an idea we just got, text a relative to get back in touch, or call our handyman to cross something that's been bugging us off our list, and on and on.

The guided journaling process can hone and polish our self-care Voice and habits continuously. It can engage our right and left brain. The harnessing of thoughts accesses the left hemisphere of the brain, which is analytical, linear, and logical. While our left brain gets organized, our right brain can be free to do what it does best—create, get the big picture, and feel around for what's right.

Along with connecting with our GPS, I believe connecting the two processes together is one of the most important things we can do to develop our trained intuition; the connection masters that Voice inside of us, helping us to discern all the data coming in, including miracle data, steering our lives with a *very powerful* compass.

Guided journaling removes our mental blocks, and allows us to use more of our brainpower to better understand our Selves and the world we're living, learning, loving, and leaving a legacy in. The process is quite amazing at getting the noise out of our mind and leaving the space remaining in our head clear, quiet, and calm.

Guided journaling also reduces emotional "overwhelm." When we translate a negative experience into language by writing it down, we essentially make the experience graspable, shrinking the size of the feelings down.

We learn to appreciate, become more aware and more understanding of our relationships from downloading our experiences. Guided journaling records our experiences for us to get far more out of our relationships when we harvest our thoughts. Guided journaling grows our knowing within our time with Joy.

When we go through and harvest our wisdom and knowledge, we can make new journal entries from old ones, because we grow and learn and gain better perspectives from the sea of "letters" we've unknowingly written to our Selves. We can evolve our intuition manual.

We can add those new entries to our updated library of wisdom, *now* knowing they will be letters to comfort and empower our future Self.

I've been journaling a long, long time. But I had to do a lot of *guided* journaling before I got to the point where I could see, let alone clear out, whatever was bugging me, then grow my time with Joy.

Now, in a matter of two or three sentences, I'm like, "Yep, I see where we're going here; that's not happening, we're going here instead."

It takes practice. And it has nothing to do with the actual length of time we journal. It has to do with the *intentional* process of journaling, and training our mind, training our body, training our spirit, to catch things quicker so we can accelerate our progress of more Joy, less stress.

For my entire life, I have asked my Self to guide me in my journals. Journal after journal, I would enter my thoughts, my dreams, my problems onto the paper, and always ask my Voice to guide me.

GUIDE ME is my acronym for Gather Understanding In Doing Everything Miraculous and Enthusiastic.

I like this acronym because it describes exactly what I am doing in my journals and what I am asking for in my life.

I have experienced an insane number of miracles in my life, so I always look for more miracles in everything I do and experience. I have also grown up with a rock-solid knowing of my Voice, so I seek to rely on the enthusiastic assurance I receive from my GPS to direct me through everything I do.

I feel like I have a perpetually miraculous life as a result of my constant commitment to learning what my strong insight has to teach me of the transcendent and inexplicable through my experiences.

Approaching our journals, our spirit, with the reverence of sitting in the company of a wisdom master, will open us up to *respect* the guidance of what we *say*.

Once we receive guidance, and we master knowing, then we do what we have been guided to, across everything we do, and everyone we are being guided with.

Then we embrace the miracles that result. Then we lean on, sit in, and sleep with our enthusiastic *intimate* comfort of *knowing*.

Guided journaling helps us practice courageous acts in advance by rehearsing on the pages what our spirit directs us to do.

The Voice is continuously strengthened through the muscle of spiritual courage floating off the pages of exercised practice into manifestations across our lives.

Guided journaling helps us to take apart our dream, piece by peace, and get the data we need to get it entirely done in a way that fulfills us the most.

When we record our progressive successes, our journals become intuition manuals that show us our full shares of the Greater Good that we've earned through our efforts and open-heartedness.

Through the strength of our Voice, what we have accomplished inside our journals has now gotten us ready for the world...to enjoy the manifestation of our Voice beyond the pen and paper.

We are able to step into a whole new world of Joy every time we finish journaling. Then our miraculous and enthusiastic *Joy* becomes the Intuition Manual we rely on to live, love, learn, and leave a legacy.

If the purpose in our living is to attend
to our own distinctive spirit,
and the character of our loving is
our lone fingerprint on the world,
then maybe the grace in our healing
is as unique as we are.

You Are Not Bound by the Hands of Time

(Another journey through my journals …)

I don't want to be here.

Today, I want to be anywhere but here…and now. Today, I am being forced to acknowledge a profound, piercing, and personal milestone. I have been unwillingly saddled with a realization that I have to accept in my life: I'm in a lot of pain.

And the burden of accepting this pain is being etched into my soul; it's changing my cells as we speak. All the while, denial has been raging within me, pacing with a ferocious energy, daring the world to be real, threatening the unimaginable if time doesn't rewind itself— right now.

But all I can feel is the hurt from this pain. And as much as I try to fight its presence, there's a complete indifference hell-bent on penetrating my body.

It's invading my limbs; it's making its way down around the tips of my fingers and up over the tips of my ears, leaving behind only numbness. It's forcing its way through every mile of my blood, and now it has gathered enough power to inject this new reality straight into the core of my being.

And my heart has become enormous from the weight of it all.

I can feel its bold rhythm dwindling to a faint throb. My vision is clouded over from spilling so many tears. I am opening my mouth to take a deep breath, but instead, the rawness of my grief is settling into my lungs, flooding me with despair. And this despair is wrapping me in its isolation, blocking my ability to see or hear or feel any compassion that comes my way.

Today, I would like to know: How on earth will I ever transcend this pain? Even as I seek to find solace within my journals, even as I am pouring my soul onto these pages in a desperate attempt to release all that lies within me, all I can feel is the pressure of time weighing down on me, stirring me to hurry up and *finish* this.

In the past, I have managed to gather enough power and wisdom to transcend the profound pain that I have had in my life...

But *this pain*...accepting *this pain* will be a work of art for me.

This is surrendering "on steroids."

I realize I should ask for help, but what I really want to do is just disappear into myself. I am hoping that the time spent in these journals will somehow lead me out of the darkness.

But I am finding I cannot think my way out of this pain. My mind has spent some time now trying to form some kind of connection or reasoning, trying to understand what's happened to me...but instead, cobwebs are spinning between my thoughts, leaving me profoundly alone and uncomprehending.

How do I use a mind that's too exhausted to help me?

How will I find my way out of the darkness? I am eclipsed by this pain. I am being forced to live so sharply and pointedly inside this very moment that I see *nothing* beyond. Inside I am empty. Inside I am sitting in nothingness, and the space all around and in between empty is *empty*. I feel like I'm not even sitting in the darkness—I am *beyond* it.

I used to believe that the gift of my emotions and my mind would teach me how I am feeling and reveal what I am thinking. But right now my pain feels bottomless. All that's being revealed to me of beyond so far is…*nothing*. All my intuitive senses seem to have been destroyed in the explosion.

My willpower to find my way through feels weary and worn-out. My senses feel like they have permanent imprints of the pain, and the pain seems to have a temporary power over me that is independent of what I choose to think or feel. My body feels like it has trauma attached to it that is independent of my will. I feel like I need to be alone and hide because I've become so exhausted from this pain. The pain seems to have the power to take me down to where *nothing* is and keep me there, but I am unwilling to stay there.

But right now, the belief that there's a strong woman in me that *will* find her way back home feels like a hysterical joke. The belief that any wisdom *will* come through for me, along with any hope of Joy that *will* reveal itself to me, feels like it's been thrown into the abyss.

I try to reconnect with my self-care habit of guided journaling, but then I think, How can I choose the practice of any contemplation when I feel like I have no *will* left to choose with?

What tools will I use to restore myself, if all I can feel is *nothing*?

It feels as if my vast world has suddenly become cellular. My hands, eyes, and ears are all affected. The tools I'm using to listen, to see, and to reach out for help feel inadequate. The life that I can still feel and see and hear is so miniscule. Whatever help might be available trying to break through to me needs to be microscopic to enter into my world, to enter through the solid barrier of my pain. Whatever relief life offers to me must be invisible to the naked eye, because I seem to be completely blind to its assistance right now.

This feels completely *beyond* me. it feels beyond my capability to fight against this intrusive, painful reality, and any attempt to restore my Self to a semblance of peace and Joy is just not happening right now.

Even if I could summon the courage to go where the pain will lead me to transcend it, then what? Remember how to recover Joy once I get there—when I have no mind to remember with? And what if I really *go there*? If I go all the way to where the pain takes me, I am afraid; will I even make it back?

And what's eventually beyond for me? Who am I to be beyond this? Right now, all I see of *beyond* is more pain. I want to know *what's beyond that.*

Not knowing what might be *beyond* is producing an anxiety of galactic proportions. Its view, its possibilities aren't on my radar. *Beyond* seems invisible, empty and black, and the inability to move out of this personal hell feels as frightening as can be.

All I can see ahead of me is this pain in my life. Every time I try to rejoin the world, the blinding colors of life are continuing on as if absolutely nothing has changed. And I am reminded of how I have been left alone with this pain inside of me, how I feel like absolutely no one on the face of this earth can climb inside and experience exactly what I am feeling. And I am reminded of the deepest aspect of my pain, that it feels like it's my burden alone to bear...all mine.

I look to see where there is *less* pain beyond this. I need to see... how do I get there? Do I lie down to rest and wait to recover and risk never getting up again? Or do I get up and keep going and risk killing my Self with exhaustion? Neither seems to be a choice because I know either way the pain stays within. It's not out there; it's inside of me.

Sometimes it seems all that's left for me in the rubble is life with pain.

Life with pain. If I am to consider this, if I am to understand this correctly, I have two choices: I can either remain in a stalemate, in a standstill at war with pain, or I can spend time with Joy, healing and restoring and transcending my life beyond the pain.

Regardless of how hard I try to be rid of it on my own, I have come to the understanding, I need my Greater Power System to put an end to this pain.

I can push and prod all I want, but I'm not getting it out the door without help.

I'm beginning to see that if I am to go beyond this very moment, I must tap into my Greater Power System's resources, which I realize is going to take some of my time and energy. And in the meantime, I must simplify my world while I take the time and rebuild the energy that I need to eradicate this pain.

This means that if I am to go on living, loving, learning, and leaving a legacy, I must be patient as I build my strength to take on the added weight of my temporary burden. This means I must stop more frequently to rest and recover as I do my job to make my Self whole again.

~

Well now, it's been a while.

I have spent time with my Greater Power System, receiving the help I need. I have spent some time with Joy.

I can see beyond now. I have been quite thorough in my efforts to restore my Self and have been able to eradicate time spent with pain.

I was hauled behind my pain at first, with my hands and my feet and my heart bound, unable to get up. I was tied and dragged through the days. But with the help of my Greater Power System, I woke up one morning and realized that the pain had slowed down, it had gotten tired...

and I had gotten stronger, much *much* stronger.

So how did I actually go from being dragged behind the pain to standing up beside it? How was I able to untie the ropes and take that first step? How did I allow my heart to join with Joy bit by bit, let the miracles change me, let the peace fill me, let new beginnings become a continuous lifeline for my soul?

With the help of my Greater Power System providing me with *enough* time with Joy.

They gave me a gift, a miraculous *grace period* with which I could eradicate the pain and instead breathe in *enough* Joy in my life.

The grace of time with Joy helped my sharpened senses to focus on one very small moment at a time; it helped me to receive each new Joyful moment as it came. Each miniscule moment carried within it all the possibilities of the world—and it also contained the miracle data I used to heal my Self with.

It contained the least amount of work I needed to navigate to get the most amount of Joy out of my life.

Time with Joy showed me that my healing is personal and it requires a reconstruction of unique and raw materials. Time with Joy taught me to respect the need of the human body to rebuild as it needs to, to respect the importance of pouring Joy back into my life.

I have not been reassembled, mended as I once was. I have been rebuilt, my soul and I, from the inside out, from the invisible to the visible.

I realize I was able to let the pain heal over time with Joy rather than let the pain become a permanent piece of me. I realize pain didn't have to *become* me...because I know I am made of something that's much more than pain. Because I believe I am much, much more than I could ever begin to understand.

I have noticed that time spreads the pain out, diluting its imposing presence. And pain that has had time to sit and rest will eventually wither away and be less oxygen-depriving.

Time with Joy is the most powerful pain eradicator there is. I have eradicated the pain, not because I *think* I am strong enough and not because I *feel* like I am strong enough, but because the pain is *gone*.

As a result, I *know* I am strong enough.

And after so much time, I have learned something profound: This hasn't been about the process of digging through the pain to get to my soul; it's been about *letting the grace of time with Joy deliver my soul to me.*

My healing is not a destination…or a number on a clock or a date on the calendar. It's *beyond* that. It's a journey of time with Joy, a boundless journey. There is no allotted amount of time to heal; there is no need to *finish* in a given amount of time. I can take all the time I need. And time is the space between this moment and the next. Space—with room enough to breathe.

I just need to *take my time with Joy* and *own* the Joy in my life.

If I need time to sit with the pain, then I need to take it and really *sit* with it, own the time I take with it. If I need the time to feel the heartbeat of my life, then I need to take it and really *feel* it, own the time I take feeling it. If I need time with Joy to enlighten more of my day, then I need to take it and really *be* with Joy, own the time I take with Joy's company.

The pain is no longer my enemy, and more importantly, it is no longer my driver. My Greater Power System has provided me with the tools I use to allow the grace of time with Joy to help me halt the pain that was in the front seat and allow Joy to take the wheel instead.

I am able to choose now; my life is filled with Joy that grows by the day.

I have chosen to participate in my life, and I have no need to try and kick my pain to the curb. The pain has ceased being a passenger; it is no longer in the vehicle.

Joy drives me now. Now we just ride through time across the gorgeous countryside. I have so much Joy visible in my rearview, reminding me of where I come from, where I've been, and in my windshield, continuously curating my experiences to spend *more* time with Joy.

~

Author's note:

My first experience with profound pain came the summer I turned thirteen, when my dad died. I remember him being in the hospital a short time, and my family and me visiting him frequently.

One day I came home from tennis lessons and found my brothers and my mom sitting around the kitchen table. She looked up at me with this pained expression as I came through the door. I was totally unprepared when she painfully announced, "Your father's gone."

My family's faces spoke of a grief much larger than her words. It frightened me and I ran outside to escape from it. I was sitting on the grass when my oldest brother, Phil, came out and sat down beside me. He grabbed my hand and said, "Anne, Dad isn't here anymore, but I am...I will be here for you."

It hit me then—what Mom was *really* saying to me.

For a while I was numb, and it took time for me to realize that Dad wasn't ever coming home from the hospital. I missed my dad (I still do), but somehow I seemed to quickly return to the business of being a kid.

It was made significantly easier because Phil lived next door. He very much filled in the unfinished father role that Dad had left behind. He and his wife took me everywhere with his five boys, and he never made me feel like I was a burden. I seemed to survive the impact of the pain with minimal scars…or so I thought.

I think one of the gifts of experiencing my dad's death as a child is that the pain didn't consume me. There was some built-in mechanism that shielded me from feeling the loss so intensely.

Not so when you become an adult.

I was twenty-one when Phil died. This time was different. I was much older…and there was much more history with him—he being the one I had looked up to as I received many years of his comfort and guidance.

He had been sick for quite a while, but it shocked me the day I was instructed to get to the hospital because he didn't have much time left. When I got there, my sister-in-law emphasized, "Go in and say good-bye…but don't expect any response, he's heavily medicated."

So I went in, not knowing what to expect or what to do. But as he lay there unresponsive, breathing shallowly, I squeezed his hand and all I could think to say was, "It's okay, Phil…You can go…I will be here for your kids."

I flinched when he squeezed my hand back.

I think I left shortly after—and I don't remember the three-hour drive home. Later on that night, my second-oldest brother, Marcel, came through the door and said, "Anne, Phil's with Dad."

We cried and hugged each other, and after some time he asked if I was okay—he needed to go home to be with his family. I told him I was fine.

But as I sat on the couch, all alone in the house, I could feel myself go numb. I could feel the pain spreading inside me. I got up and went down into the basement to be really alone with my pain. I curled up into a ball and heaved huge sobs for hours upon hours. Every time I thought I'd emptied myself of the pain, thinking I was past it, the reality

of Phil's passing would hit me again and the pain would start all over…
more waves of sobbing, more waves of grief.

This went on for most of the night. I think I was determined not
to exit that cellar until I could be rid of that pain for good. But all I
accomplished was extreme exhaustion.

I eventually came upstairs and went straight to bed.

The days and weeks and months passed, and I realized my life
would never be the same. It was very difficult to watch my mother
come to terms with one of her own children departing this life before
she did. It was very difficult to watch my newly widowed sister-in-law
raise five boys on her own.

I stayed close by her and the boys as I'd promised, doing what little
a young twenty-something could do to help Phil's kids get on with the
business of being kids (as I had some experience with this myself).

After Phil died, I remember thinking, I've surely met life's pain
quota now. I have learned what is important in life and I will take very
little for granted. I've gotten thoroughly bitten by the reverence-for-life
snake, so I'm good for a while…or so I thought.

A few years later, I found out that Linda, the wife of my third-oldest
brother, Francis, was very sick.

It would be two courageous years before Linda would let go of this
life and leave behind my brother and their three children. I remember
spending many wonderful childhood summer vacations with her and
the kids. I remember feeling the loss of yet another person in my life
that I loved very much, and watching my brother work diligently to
help *his* children get on with the business of being kids.

The physical intensity of this loss was much less than my brother's because there was much less shock at the fragility of life this time
around. But there was much more depression and sadness as I spent
weeks and months coming to grips with another hole added to my life.

The pain in my life had not yet met its quota.

After Linda's death, I found myself paying extra attention to what I wanted out of my life. I found myself more exacting in my life choices, choosing carefully how I spent my time on this earth because I had learned well—life is just too precious to waste. All the pain of loss was continuously repurposing me and shaping the character of my love.

I think I have cherished the remaining relationships that are closest to me pretty conscientiously—not knowing when their time might be up. And I have lived *my* life pretty intensely, not knowing when *my* time might be up. As a result, I tend to exist on a daily basis at a depth that most people gloss over.

I used to live with the fear of death and loss in all its forms…chasing me, nipping at my heels. Actually, I don't think it's so much the *fear* of all this pain, but the *reality* of it that was seared into my bones, that drove home the possibility that I might not live my life to its fullest or that I might not cherish all that life had given me.

No regrets, no limits. That's been my motto.

When I was thirty-nine, pain revisited me again when Mom died. We had a six-month heads-up this time, and my grieving process was very different from the others in the family. Mom and I had spent so much time jointly working through all the other pain and losses over the years, we just seemed to continue our work together…but with way more hugs and tears.

We had many more intense conversations, trying our best to help each other embrace the painful goodbye that was just around the corner. We had an incredible six months together. She was very conscious of the pain that lay in wait for me beyond her death, and I was very conscious of the struggle with her faith in a grace that she prayed would deliver her soul when she needed it most.

After her passing, the pain felt more mature and experienced in me. I was more accepting…more calm and at peace. I gave myself plenty of time and space. No judgment or expectations of what I should be doing and how fast I should be doing it. I wasn't in a hurry. I was quite amazed, actually. I seemed to grieve much more effortlessly; I felt like I had *learned* what was beyond.

I was embracing *grace*.

For a few years after Mom's passing, I felt different than I did before her death. I remember thinking, Well, that was not so bad this time. Maybe I *have* met my quota for pain after all. Maybe I don't have to live in fear, anticipating what other burden I might have to learn to shoulder, what more pain I might have to endure. I must have this pain thing down by now…I must have *finally* spent enough time with it.

I felt like maybe I could take time to relax and not be so intense—not have such sharpened senses. Maybe I could slow down and take my time with all that I dreamed of…maybe I could do a little cruisin' through my life.

But then the day came when the pain slammed on the brakes and threw me to the curb.

I had a routine mammogram that resulted in a call to come in for a double breast biopsy. They needed to "investigate" the spots in the pictures. Deep down inside I was reeling, and on the surface were all the voices telling me "not to worry…keep a positive attitude…cross that bridge when you get to it."

(What bridge?)

I fell off the cliff when the telephone rang. I was freefalling at the *reality* of my own impending death. With my family history, I wasn't living in "if"; I was immersed in "when."

I spent the entire week numb, deaf, and blind to the world around me because of my terror. *I haven't finished with my life yet.* I spent the entire week right back down in the basement of my mind. When no one was around, I would cry…trying to *will* the possible, painful reality away.

In the space of one momentous ring, all the work I had done to master this class of life with pain had disintegrated.

Clearly, I had more work to do.

When I lay on that gurney waiting to go into surgery, I came completely unglued. I wept uncontrollably as the years of pain and loss I was trying to outrun caught up with me.

I remember the kind and compassionate nurses assuring me that many women go through this procedure and come out perfectly fine. But they didn't know anything about *me*. They didn't know what I knew. They didn't know that I knew *exactly* what kind of pain life could dish out.

$\sim$

In the end, the biopsies were normal.

That night, I slept normally. That week, my life went back to normal. But I've realized…I will never be "normal."

That was made clear when I was on the inside with my *pain*…and the nurses were on the outside with their *life*. I remember feeling very alone as I witnessed their discomfort at my accumulated grief. They weren't cold to it, just uncomprehending of the *depth* of it.

Which is why I ended up going back through all my pain to write this. I wanted to revisit the journey through my fear of death and all the different experiences I've had of pain and loss. And I have found that the journey I have taken from shock to acceptance to Joy…has been purely the work of my Greater Power System providing me the grace of *time with Joy*.

Time spent with Joy is what I needed enough of, not more time with pain. I needed to be *informed* by my pain, and not nurture the processing of it to the point I became stuck in an eddy of pain. And I needed to be able to *nurture* my Joy and not just be informed of it, so I would fully absorb its miraculous properties.

At one point, when I was younger, I remember my brother Pat telling me not to grab onto pain and live life going from one pain to the next, but instead to grab onto Joy and go from one Joy to the next. That stuck with me, and I've made sure to do exactly that.

Pain is universal, but the healing of it is *very* personal and unique. Not all of my pain has had the same intensity, or the same longevity, or the same effect on my life. Some of my pain has taken me longer to heal from than others, but *all* have been transformed with *enough* time spent with Joy (like I have much less fear of my own certain death because I have seen what's "beyond"; I have finished so many pieces of me in so many ways with Joy, I get more satiated by the day).

My family, my friends, and my community have all been instrumental with getting me completely through every single pain and loss I have had by filling me up with Joy, helping me to empty the pain from my life through enough time with Joy.

The depth and breadth of the deep Joy delivered to me by all those around me continues to prove to me just how precious *I* am … to show me just how much *my* Joy *matters*.

I feel it all day long every day as I write and paint and teach and entrepreneur and play.

Healing over time with Joy is a journey that is intensely personal. It is crucial that we reach out when we are in pain, or experiencing loss. It is crucial that we help our Selves to heal from pain, restore our Selves after a loss, and evolve our lives with Joy. It is crucial we give our Selves enough time with Joy to master the self-care habits we need to live our greatest lives and to share our greatest Selves to evolve those around us.

I've learned now that I am never alone in my journey, my Greater Power System has my back. I know now that time spent with Joy heals, restores, and grows every piece of me *beyond*, with new Joy constantly being delivered to me.

With the help of my Greater Power System, time with Joy has repeatedly delivered to me a fully complete yet honed life, filled with memories and dreams to cherish now.

I love my life. The Joy I receive continually raises my spirit.

Each day begins with me in Joyful expectation. The day passes with Joy raising my spirit, pouring miracles into my life. Each day ends with Joy fully expressed in me.

I am immensely grateful for the Joy that has been shared with me. "Time heals all wounds" is easy to misunderstand. I learned from my journey with my Greater Power System, that it is time with Joy that heals all wounds.

Ascensions

When I was three, I contracted German measles. My mother believed I had had the shot, but there was a slip-up with the paperwork at the doctor's office, and when the disease made its rounds, I caught it.

I had a very high fever, and as a result I lost 40–45% of my hearing, particularly in the range of human speech tones.

I have had hearing aids since then but have struggled to hear many conversations, sounds, and words over the decades.

Hearing aids are costly, and I took good care of each set I had, so I could go as long as possible without upgrading them.

When my mother was dying and getting her financial affairs in order, she was adamant that I get new hearing aids and that she'd pay for them.

At the time, the ones I had were frequently breaking down, and I often went without them, resulting in her frustration with me missing out on so much communication.

In her last months, while she was alive, I was too busy raising my children, running the businesses, and doing hospice care for her, to take the time to get fitted for new hearing aids.

When she passed and I received my inheritance, it was one of the first things I did.

The day I went home with the first new digital version of hearing aids ever was one of the most memorable, miraculous days of my life.

That day, as I walked out of Mark's (my hearing aid specialist) office, it was raining. I ran to my vehicle, jumped in, and shook off the wetness and froze in my seat.

I was 40 years old, and for the first time in my life, I could hear rain.

The rain produced such a beautiful, musical sound as the drops randomly danced on my roof and windows…I sat in the parking lot, mesmerized by the *sound* for such a long time. Tears poured down my face, matching the water running in rivers down my windshield.

I drove home crying.

I was in such awe of the sound of something so simple, so unnoticed by so many, and of the power my new hearing aids had, to bless me with the glorious music I was now privy to.

The morning after I got my new hearing aids, I went to leave the house and was stopped in my tracks at the bottom of my steps. I couldn't figure out what the whistling, whooshing sound was that I was hearing.

I was told it was the wind blowing through the leaves on the trees in my yard. I couldn't believe the sound that it made—I had no idea such a sound existed.

I stood there for a bit with my face lifted to the sunshine and closed my eyes as I listened to the rustling of the wind moving through the leaves.

When I opened my eyes, I noticed that, as the leaves moved, I also felt that same soft, dry whisper moving in and across my body, except now I could hear it. I stood there just feeling the breeze on my skin and listening to it as I watched the leaves dance to the air…for almost a half hour.

My auditory miracles continued, every day, all day for the weeks and months following.

For over a year afterward, I had to retrain my brain to label, sort, and file every new sound I was hearing that I had never heard before.

I heard my first chipmunk scurrying through trees. I learned all the different sounds of birds. I heard water babbling in a brook clearer than ever before. I heard entire conversations for the first time.

A whole new world was opening up to me.

The first time my feet crunched across the rocks on my driveway had me stopping in glee like a new baby walking for the first time.

I was enthralled with the crunch my shoes were making with each footstep. And I literally just walked all over my driveway…stepping, dragging, stomping my shoes across the rocks, listening to the newest, coolest sound *ever*, and laughing at the sound of it all, including what my own clearer-than-ever laughter sounded like.

For at least a year after getting my new hearing aids, I was exhausted from forming all these connections between my ears and my brain, training me in all the newest additions to my auditory world.

In some environments, there were times when I had a new sound every few minutes, and I was nonstop asking those around me what the noises were so I could stop being so distracted by them.

Strange noises stopped me while I was doing things, and new sounds trumped my concentration. Unheard-of auditory nuances interrupted me continuously.

As a result of the new technology in hearing aids that I now enjoy, I have since grown to feel more included in the world I'm in.

I feel included in society. I feel included in conversations and whispers. I feel included in the lyrics to music and dialogue in movies.

THE INTUITION MANUAL: BOOK 1

I feel included in nature. I feel included in the ocean waves and babbling streams. I feel included in the fluttering of partridges and the drumming of woodpeckers.

To all those engineers and technicians responsible for the evolution of hearing aids, *thank you.*

I still have limitations with my hearing, especially in large crowds—I still do a great deal of watching people speak to discern the similar sounds within the vowels and consonants that I hear.

In any size group, I still instinctively read body language to discern the tones of the words and the meaning of the sentences and questions that are spoken.

I still can't hear high tones of human speech very well. But with my new hearing aids, I now can make more sense of the sounds I *do* hear, to go with the sense of sight I so heavily rely on to "hear" someone.

I find the human senses fascinating. What we lack in one area sometimes becomes heightened in another area, like when I rely on my sight to augment my handicapped hearing.

I was very young when I learned to "read" the lips of my family and friends, and somewhere along the way, I mastered reading the body language of people, as well.

With my sense of hearing impaired, I find my other senses are more exercised. Compared to a lot of people around me, it seems my senses of sight, smell, taste, and touch are quite sensitive.

The Joy that is elevated in me from the restoration of so much of my hearing loss has been wonderful. With my ongoing auditory evolution, I am able to use my raised Joy to expand my Self through my community, to scale up the progress in my dreams, to exponentially increase my peace, and fully detail the satisfaction in my life.

When we reach the pinnacle of Joy as we see, smell, feel, taste, and hear new transcendent information that takes us beyond what we previously knew, we experience an ascension into heaven on earth.

When we experience the heightened *sense of Joy* in us within a transcendent event, we realize, "Ahh, so *this* level of Joy is what's possible for me," and our newfound intimate *knowing* that *that* Joy exists, soars our spirit.

The shortest, most amazing route to heaven on earth is through the joy experienced by our senses that include our sense of Spirit.

There are all kinds of information that are discerned with our sense of Spirit in conjunction with our five physical senses.

We sense Joy in our spirit when we ingest Joy in our human world.

We don't just see, smell, feel, taste, or hear to gather and respond to the information that gets combined and interpreted by our human brain. We have a spiritual sense that runs through all of that, that tells us what brings us Joy and what doesn't.

And with that spiritual sense, we have the power to evolve our sense of Joy.

The body and mind have their human limits, but within those limits, our spirit can transcend us with Joy. Our ascension to heaven on earth requires both us and our Greater Power System to heal, and hold, and honor, and heighten the Joy in our life.

We do this not only by not shunning the sense of Joy experienced through the spirit, but with heightening our sense of Spirit with each other.

We can refuse to allow anyone to shun what brings us Joy. And we can heal, and hold, and honor, and heighten what Joy we already possess.

Language carries tremendous power from one person to another and from us to our Selves. Language with Hoover Dam power, Niagara Falls power, hurricane-force wind power, volcanic eruption power, tidal wave power...can have either negative or positive effects on our ascensions.

Obviously, we would do well to not tolerate abuse of each other or our Selves with language that causes power outages in the spirit.

Across the physical, emotional, mental, and social bodies there is a language that humans can "read" that can contain zero auditory noise. It's just visual, yet *vocal*, visceral language spoken throughout the body, without uttering a sound, that is heard by the spiritual body.

Modern society sometimes has struggles with body language literacy. Sometimes the person living in the body isn't "home" enough to "read" what the spiritual body would like to tell them.

Sometimes we are quite busy, with less time for live in-person community. Sometimes we are behind our technology, with less live in-person communication. Sometimes we are quite tired, with less energy for live in-person connection.

Body language is entirely separate from the spoken language but is "read" along with the spoken language. If body language is missing from our methods of communication, we handicap ourselves with the training needed to "read" Joy. When we are trained in reading spiritual body language, we become super human cap*able.*

We recognize authentic people as being authentic when their spoken language and body language are saying the same thing. We *know* they're being authentic because their behavior is consistently trustworthy.

We recognize joyful people as being joyful when their spoken language and body language both have the "Voice" of Joy laced through them. We *know* they're exuding Joy because their sharing of it is consistently inclusive.

The ascension of our spirit with our Voice of Joy is provided for, nurtured, and protected with the knowing that develops when information is seen, smelled, felt, tasted, and heard by our spirit.

The Joy in our spirit directs our knowing through those five senses in "reading" and making sense of new information. The language that travels from one body to another is all read by our spirit.

Like when we "feel" someone's intention or there's a sense of understanding that someone conveys to us.

There's a sense of patience, or a sense of passion people *have*. There's a sense of enthusiasm people *bring*. There's a sense of light we *experience* in people.

Then there are senses when we declare, "That makes total sense," or "that makes perfect sense."

Sometimes we have the good sense to do something "right." Sometimes we can't shake the sense that something is "wrong."

And then there's someone's unmistakable sense of humor. And of course, our sense of purpose that drives us.

Common sense includes the intuitive senses. Street sense uses our sense of fear. A false sense is caught by our inner sense.

And on and on we all try to make sense of everything we take in. The sense we need most in this world is our sense of Joy to take it all in.

When we experience Joy anywhere in one sense, it travels throughout our body via our raised spirit. Through the ascension of our spirit, the rest of our body gets to hitch a ride on the Joy train.

The environment that our senses live, love, learn, and leave a legacy in needs to be full of Joy. It is crucial that what we take in with our senses day in and day out doesn't mute our wonderment. That the "information" we see, smell, taste, feel, or hear to make love with our world, doesn't tear down our spirit…doesn't turn down the volume of our Joy. We want the life we live to make spiritual sense. We want the time and energy we use up to make sense with our values. We want our entire lives to feel *sensual*.

Every glorious sight, fragrance, flavor, touch, sound intentionally sought out and incorporated into our environment can ascend our spirit.

When we have a space we are empowered to live in, to love in, to learn in, and to leave a legacy in, any unwanted sight, fragrance, flavor, touch, or sound can be, one by one, removed from our life in order to ascend our spirit.

These spaces can be any physical space, emotional space, mental space, or social space we are empowered to grow our Joy in, but they are all heightened with our spiritual space connecting all of these to us.

A soul that resides in a stressed space due to Joy not heightened by the five senses is a soul that is missing beautiful pieces of heaven on earth.

It is essential that we pay attention to when Spirit is communicating through our bodies with both stress *and* Joy and let stress inform us and Joy nurture us. Not the other way around.

You want to be aware of a-sense-*shuns*—when our rising to our fully connected Selves, with all our senses engaged, is shunned, with the most important sense of these being our spiritual sense.

The first task to heighten our senses, including our sense of Spirit, is to clear from our five senses negativity that shuns our sense of Spirit.

With awareness, we can sense the negative within our entire body and take steps to remove it. We can sense what is positive for us and notice when it's missing.

When we can repeatedly switch the details of a negative environment out with a positive one, the ascension of our spirit continues to climb in power within the Greater Good.

The ascension of us does not require us to hold our Self down so that others don't feel "put off" by the height of our passion.

The ascension of us does not require us to be placed as low as we can be so that when we rise up, we do not put anyone else down by the height of our Joy.

Achieving heaven on earth starts with an include-us-in-the-satisfaction paradigm, so we are able to exude Joy for others who choose to be included and satisfied with Joy, as well.

We can ascend our entire lives starting with paying attention to the five physical senses on a physical level and transform them with Joy that shows us how much we value our Selves.

In our journals, we can go through our daily life and start picking off things that don't bring us Joy, make plans, and add more and more of the things that do bring us Joy.

We can use these questions to help us:

What does our sense of self-worth smell like to us?

Does it smell like daily walks in the pine-scented forest? Like lavender pillows on our bed at night? Like candles burning in our home? Like a pie baking in the oven? Like a freshly bathed body? Like flowers on our kitchen table?

We can add what smells good to us, that makes us feel nurtured, then ascend others with our Joy from them.

What does our sense of self-worth taste like to us? Does it taste like raspberries? Daily salads? Lobsters and clams? Our favorite piece of chocolate? A welcome-home kiss?

What does our sense of self-worth feel like to us? Does it feel like silk that breathes? Like velvet? Spandex to move around in? Does it feel like massages on our skin? Like fur we love to stroke?

What does our sense of self-worth look like to us? Jeweled art? Body curves? Sharp dressing? How about clean spaces? Designs that elevate function?

What does our sense of self-worth sound like to us? Waves on the beach? Rain in the forest? Words of love for our beauty? Music that makes us move? Whispers of intimacy?

We can add what smells, tastes, feels, looks, and sounds good to us, that makes us feel nurtured, then ascend others with our Joy from them.

We can enjoy expanding our soul with this process. And keep on the lookout for more ways we and our Greater Power System can ascend each of us with our satisfaction in the life we're living, loving, learning, and leaving a legacy in.

SWAT Teams

Bullsh-t.

It's what we sometimes say when the spiritual math between someone's actions and their words consistently *doesn't add up* in a relationship.

It's when our spirit recognizes that something is "off" with a person's body language and we recognize their repetitive negative behavior as intentional abuse.

The "breaking of the bread"—the shared Joy within the relationship experiences—seems to frequently taste bad. The person seeks to erode our half of the bread again and again with their abusive grooming of what we believe we deserve.

Their words say they simply need our help with their self-care, while their body language seeks power to control the freedom of *our* self-care.

Their words say we're fully empowered to participate in the Greater Good, while their body language seeks power to control our access to who and what brings us Joy.

Their words say we're fully included in breaking bread with Joy, while their body language seeks power to control every aspect of how that Joy is disbursed.

Their words say we have freedom with our share of generosity, while their body language seeks power to control our compassionate efforts by manipulating our empathy.

Their words say they provide for, nurture, and protect us, while their body language seeks power to control our autonomy from deep within our altruism.

To maintain our freedom when breaking bread, our spiritual intelligence has to be trained with Joy within the Greater Power System. We have to experience words and body language that are congruent, and be taught to recognize when an intentional abuser's isn't.

We have to learn to recognize when the result of consistent lack of integrity adds up to the sum of what we call spiritual violence from an intentional abuser seeking to swallow our light completely into the black hole of their needs.

And when they are in a position of power above us, our trained spirit can recognize them as an abusive higher power.

When we have been trained within our Greater Power System to recognize the imprisoning lies that get ingested by our spiritual body, we can digest the truth once we gut-check it with the GPS-verified *validity* of *our* experience.

We then can eradicate any continuing presence of an intentional abuser in our lives once every bone in our body tells us an intentional abuser's trustworthiness is total *bullsh-t*.

We can recognize when their connection with us isn't honest. Their integrity is not congruent. The *relationship* isn't *safe*.

With spiritual training, we can see the balance in the shared accounts of Joy being manipulated by them for their perpetual gain and our continuous loss—until we do the spiritual math, end the relationship, and close all our accounts with them.

Within our spirit, within our trained intuition, we can see inside their relentless demands, in their "limits" dismantling our boundaries, or within the missing math in their seemingly reasonable spiritual calculations.

We can see silent but deadly control within their body language *expecting* us to hand over more power. We can see the malicious *intent* inside their communication that sends our precious spirit a wake-up call to action.

When we use the Intuition Manual, we can see what lies beneath language and behavior. We can recognize that there is the actual trained communication within physical integrity, but there is also the trained communication inside emotional, mental, and social integrity, all filtered through our spiritual intelligence.

We recognize when there are dishonest moments our intuitive Voice sums up as insincere. We immediately spot spiritually irreconcilable language and actions.

This collective human communication, in addition to our spiritual intelligence, becomes the most powerful evolutionary algorithm we can use to solve the math of intentional abusive use of power.

With our bullsh-t radar detector fully operational, with our trained intuition fully engaged, we then *know* whether we are in the presence of an abusive higher power vs. a Greater Power System, and we can respond with correct empowering action.

We can multiply our spiritual wealth within our Greater Power System, while placing stop payments on our checks to an abusive higher power.

Whether it be in the home, the workplace, the school, the community, or the country, we may encounter an intentional abuser who operates under the guise of the Greater Good to grow their regime, rule, and reign of power to control.

Sometimes they want to watch the world burn just because… they're *hungry*.

Just because is the motto on their coin. "Just" cause is their creed. Their mission is to disintegrate and incinerate and obliterate our right to share in the bread of Joy.

When they try to bury our spirit in their bullsh-t with their attempts to steal the pieces of our independent, incalculably precious, cap*able* power away from us, when they seek to hollow out our Joy from the core of our body and soul, they remain indifferent about causing spiritual destruction and are frequently oblivious to any negative repercussions.

With an intentional abuser, the insatiable need for power to control is the only spiritual math that matters to them.

They live in a zero-sum world where they can't just win…*we also must lose*. The core of who we are must be hollowed out to feed their relentless need to acquire more power.

Intentional abusers never actually empower with the power they "dispense." Whatever empowerment we receive from them is never freely given. Ultimately, their "gift" must come back around to *them* to serve their cause.

They seek to always boomerang power back to themselves; they want us to believe we can't get Joy without *their* consent.

Intentional abusers have infallible beliefs about themselves and their cause. *They* don't make mistakes; therefore, they take no responsibility for any. They apologize, but not really. They rule the body language airwaves with the threat of *more* loss of our Joy, within their false "sharing" narrative.

They seek to make sure everyone beneath them serves their cause because their insatiable hunger demands it. They try to dictate how, what, where, when, and who is included in their personal "greater good."

They try to attack our freedom, criticize our altruism, punish our autonomy. We have no right to *volunteer* our service to their cause, because until we get out, it's mandatory. We have no right to choose our own sacrifices.

Sometimes, they require us to look them in the eye so they can see if the answer to their repeated blows of, "Did you *die* yet?" is revealed through the windows to our soul.

We are not allowed to have independence within the relationship. We are not allowed to have independence of thoughts, independence of feelings, independence of action. We are only allowed absolute identity with their cause.

It's tricky when we find our Selves in an abusive higher-powered relationship, because at first their power to control will include us in their cause just enough to charm us, to keep us going in the relationship long enough to become groomed by their veiled hunger.

Over time, in the imbalance of power, we lose the ability to express independent thought, feeling, or action within the vast reach of their control.

Over time, we are abusively trained…with our borders now defined inside *their* borders, our empowering boundaries now suppressed inside *their* boundaries.

Over time, we become monitored closely, we become restricted discreetly, and unless we do the spiritual math, we are seized unconsciously.

Over time, outside their boundaries we can *remain* abusively trained, lest they violently erupt to expand the borders of their power, when they catch us not defending their cause.

Just exploring our negative experience of the relationship is decreed as irrelevant to the mission at hand. Just expressing our negative experience of the relationship is interpreted as dissent from their authority. Just exiting our negative experience of the relationship is considered heresy against their apocryphal quest to be the only one who wins.

The false "joint" relationship isn't truly inclusive.

In an abusive higher-powered relationship, we are not empowered to remove our Selves from the "joint" obligations. We are not empowered to rid our Selves of the "joint" pain. We are not empowered to reimagine our Selves free because of the "joint" sacrifices they decree are still to be made.

We are not empowered to choose what share of the *actual* Greater Good we deserve. We are not empowered to balance the joint account.

The power to choose doesn't include us. The power to consent doesn't include us. The power to control doesn't include us. And as a result, the power to provide for, nurture, and protect *us* is denied to us.

Abusive power makes the Joy in our lives feel very hard and brittle and extremely fragile to hold onto.

Abusive power will force us to say no when our will is to say yes to Joy, and to say yes when our will is to say no to stress.

All this power to control run amok requires an alternate power to stop it—an *intuitively* trained power.

Mastery in purging, processing, and preventing intentional abuse requires training within the shelter and protection and nurturance of a trained intuitive community within a Greater Power System.

The trained intuitive community contains your SWAT team. (My best friend once coined the acronym SWAT team as the **S**h-tshow **W**ith **A**ngels **T**raining team, and it stuck with me.) Sh-tshows are temporary abusive events manufactured by intentional abusers.

A SWAT team is a team of people within our Greater Good community made up of persons of exemplary conduct or virtue, training us in all things Joy—training us with the Intuition Manual that we use to repeatedly transcend with Joy and remove temporary times of sh-tshows from our lives.

I learned a lot about how Great my community was when I was a hairdresser for twenty years. In addition to the training my family and friends provided me with, I was able to get to know a lot of people, both in my salon, day in and day out, and in their homes when I did special events and house calls. I watched entire families grow up before my eyes.

99.99% of my clients were absolutely amazing people to break bread with, and a minor few had to be removed from my client list due to their abusive behavior.

I remember once, seeing a kind, highly intelligent, independent, and very capable little boy sitting on a floor leaning over and intently playing with building blocks…concentrating hard on constructing his vision with his nimble little fingers.

After some time, he halted abruptly, leaned back, and looked at his creation in satisfaction. He started clapping his hands excitedly and sat up straight, proudly admiring his achievement as a big smile spread across his face.

We could plainly see the Joy in his eyes and hear it in his voice, and he immediately sought to share it with an adult who had just entered the room, by exclaiming, "Look what I did!"

Instead of joining in the child's Joy, this person went into a rage over something that had absolutely nothing to do with the child. He chose this moment to take it out on the little boy…shredding the child's euphoria to pieces, collapsing the ebullience in the boy's face instantly, and substituting it with shame in making "such a grave mistake."

The boy was two years old.

The man's wrath had nothing to do with the young child, but he didn't let up until he made sure his body language conveyed to that little boy that the rage was *his* fault.

He was completely immune to the boy feeling horrible about his "unacceptable" behavior and refused to accept any responsibility for his effect on the child.

All that mattered was his *desire* to rage.

As the adult kept firing at the boy, the boy's expression went from shame at his "mistake" to anger turned within. His utter helplessness to "fix his mistake" and restore the adult to any sense of peace overwhelmed him.

The light in the boy's eyes darkened, and he lashed out in anger at his just-completed creation and destroyed it.

This was a relationship that, over time, from the repetition of abuse, taught the boy that it was dangerous to ever share his Joy with this man.

The man was incapable of sharing in Joy because he had little of it himself. He was consumed with the black hole of his deprivation and his need to repeatedly fill it. (Black holes skew the spiritual math of Joy way out of balance.)

I noticed a pattern with him. Whenever someone else had Joy, he perceived that he was owed payment for it in some form. In his mind, he was making the most sacrifices in the spiritual math because he was always hungry, so therefore, their Joy also belonged to *him* in some way.

The child knew he was safer if he kept his Joy deeply hidden whenever he was in this man's presence.

As the child grew up, he stayed far away from any chance of being attacked, by not drawing attention to his Joy. He shied away from drawing any attention to his satisfaction. He made sure he was never too happy in case he offended.

As an adult, he transcended these times of sh-tshows. He was able to fully gain power to control the sharing of his Joy without abuse, with training from his SWAT team members.

In another event, there was an exceptionally smart, capable, responsible, eager-to-please young girl temporarily sharing a room with an adult who demanded silence in the entire space as he watched the TV.

She was playing quietly by herself, enjoying her toys on the table in front of her on the other side of the room. After some time, she absent-mindedly started singing happily to herself.

The adult abruptly paused the TV, stomped over to her, and went into a rage over her interruption. The sudden attack ripped her concentration from her imaginary world, and her face went from complete effusive Joy to wide-eyed horror.

He berated her, bringing her to tears, hounding her for an answer to the question of *why* she was making noise.

She sat crumpled in defeat when she couldn't give him a satisfactory answer. In her young mind, all she could come up with was, "I don't know."

He kept at her, attacking her every answer, dissecting every "excuse," causing her to feel angry at her own helplessness in making a "mistake."

He led her to only two choices for an acceptable answer: Either she was stupid, or she was intentionally trying to abuse him. The choice of simply being innocently unaware was removed.

Whenever she was in the company of this adult and had to share the space with him, she worked hard to be hyper focused to try and not make any mistakes. Over time, she became terrified of being caught unaware and making an error in his presence.

She learned to stay out of his way and keep the Joy in her experiences private.

When she grew up, she followed her Voice and grew her power to express Joy without abuse. She mastered her self-care habits to allow herself to freely shine the best of her Self out into the world. She actively sought out members of her SWAT team to get trained in Joy and transcend those sh-tshow experiences.

~

We cannot underestimate the power of the SWAT teams in our community to restore our full power to us. Our transcendence from times of sh-tshows to lives full of Joy is so much healthier and faster with their help.

In a relationship with an abusive dominating power, the relationship is either vertical or appears "horizontal," the power structure being hierarchal with only one party receiving enough Joy.

In a relationship within a Greater Power System, the power structure is both vertical *and* horizontal, with the power structure being cooperative and inclusive, with each party taking turns, each party constantly balancing their Selves equitably with the other, each continually receiving full experiences of Joy.

SWAT team members train us in this.

The power to control within the Greater Good requires spiritual maturity through experience with Joy. The power to control needs our Intuition Manual to govern our control of power.

SWAT team members train us in this.

The power to control need not be equal between a person and a small child for the safety of the child, but the growing child must have *meaningful equality of opportunity* to train up in the inclusion of Joy within the Greater Good.

Again, SWAT team members train us in this.

A spirit being raised up to maturity requires that the spirit reside in a community using their Intuition Manual to train them to own their own power fully intact and operational within the Greater Good, in order to empower Joy in everyone.

We can all train up a spirit in breaking bread; we can all be angels training with Joy. We can provide guidance as to how to grow progressively all the way through to spiritual maturity with a SWAT team's help, with the community's inclusive Joy shared as examples.

Additionally, a spirit raised within a Greater Power System learns the spiritual math they need to ensure the sum of their Joy consistently adds up in all their relationships.

If they find themselves temporarily in a relationship with an abusive higher power, they rely on their strong spiritual training to put an end to the relationship.

They know when there's an inequitable difference in the spiritual equation, and they do what it takes to halt the abuse.

And they know the power to institute *greater* self-care habits requires them to *continue* getting trained with Joy. The discernment of their decisions is honed with the training they get in the full joy they receive within the Greater Good.

A Greater Power System guides us to act from our power fully matured and secured, so all parties can embrace and express and evolve Joy.

Our spiritual body needs to dine on someone's Joy with all of our physical, emotional, mental, and social senses, while being trained in what bullsh-t to eliminate as well.

A SWAT team hones the differences in experiences between an abusive higher power seeking to drain our Joy and our GPS guiding us with our body language as to how, when, where, and with whom to dine on the bread of Joy, in peace.

A SWAT team can help us get further upstream, away from abuse, with awareness of Joy in our body as we make positive, proactive, progressive choices toward more Joy.

Our SWAT team members help us to learn the origin of a stomach sick with dread vs. the origin of a stomach full of excited butterflies, so we can eliminate the source of the bullsh-t of the former and multiply the sources of Joy in our lives with the latter.

Before we can break bread with others, we must also be free to break bread with our Selves first…we must also be free to provide for, nurture, and protect our self-care choices.

And we must get training in how big the Greater Good loaf is so we can understand what we deserve before we partake in our "half" of the bread.

And the people we hang with need to be empowered with intimate knowledge of how big their loaf is as well, so we don't let them go without in order to serve us.

And to receive training in spiritual intelligence, we need leaders who choose to share with us all that is spiritually positive for them. We need them to share what breaking the bread of Joy looks like when neither party goes hungry.

We need leaders who have the power to control their lives enough to teach us how to experience Joy that includes us. So we can put the pieces of our Selves together, from our leaders' examples, after we have experienced aloneness, hunger, or disconnection from abuse. So we can experience integrity and intimacy from acts of self-care that include our Joy. So we can use our share of the bread to *rise* within the Greater Good.

We need leaders whose spiritual intelligence raises us, by raising our spirits within our homes, our workplaces, our schools, our communities, and our countries.

When ingesting stress, we can choose to process, then purge it so Joy comes out of our efforts instead of stress. Of course, the less stress we have to process and purge, the more time we have with Joy.

Hence the need for SWAT team members within the Greater Power

System to lead the community in eradicating unnecessary stressful relationships.

There's a positive, proactive, progressive circle of life when a spirit spends time with Joy. When we eat the bread of Joy, we digest the life it gives us, and that aliveness comes out in some evolved form of spiritual fertilizer for others to plant their dreams in.

By our example, others can learn they do not have to endure remaining imprisoned by stress-filled abusers seeking to burn down the spirit of humanity.

To experience the satiation of peace within our shared relationships, we need Joy to transcend us from the outside in, feeding Joy to our spirit from the inside out, which then empowers us to pay our Joy forward.

When we have connected our satiated spiritual Selves altruistically to our homes, our workplaces, our schools, our communities, and our countries, we have multiplied the wealth of the shared Joy and eliminated the bullsh-t.

If you can be transparent as you surrender to your divine light,
you will make visible your spirit.
If you can be courageous and set free your soul's joy,
you will make known your worth.
If you can trust that this is the work you came here to do,
you will make peace with your life.

Greatness Is in the Eye of the Beholder

(Another journey through my journals…)

I'm going to die.

I don't know when or how, but I most certainly will die.

And if death is supposed to teach me to live, then I want to pay close attention in class.

I don't want to take my life for granted. I don't want to spend another day imprisoned by the lack of depth and meaning in my life, and I don't want to waste another minute of it feeling small and insignificant.

I dream of becoming somebody great. I look at great people I admire, and I have stage envy. I seem to crave a bigger life, a bigger audience. I want to feel like I'm someone important. I want to do work that ripples far and wide so I can feel like I'm doing something significant.

If I died in my sleep tonight, I believe I would be leaving much of me unfinished. And I don't want to die feeling invisible, missing my chance to leave my mark on this world.

For most of my life, while I've been searching for what I truly came here to do, I've been seeking the reflection of my worth in the eyes of humanity. While I've been searching high and low, combing the planet for the outlet to plug my Self into, I've been trying to make a connection that would truly light up my soul.

For some time now, I've been wrestling with this Voice inside of me. I've been resisting this unschooled, undeniable, uprising passion within me.

I've been *afraid*.

I keep coming back to this unrelenting Voice, insisting that the Greatness I seek…*lies within*.

I believe *Life* has been calling me. And I have finally decided to answer it.

And since I haven't been able to consistently find the answer in the world *outside* of me, I've decided to find it in the world *inside* of me.

I've decided it's time to find the eternal beauty within myself and not look for it in the mirror of society. It's time to embrace the truth of all that I am and not wait in vain for someone else to recognize its value.

It's time to *be* an inspiration of hope, to *use my life* as an example of the possibilities that lie within all of us, and not spend my days in profound invisibility as I wait for the next person to come along and emancipate *me*.

I am going to release all the Joy that lies within me. I am going to paint the world in beautiful, bold, brilliant strokes. I am going to ride through the countryside waving the radiant colors of *my* beauty, *my* truth—my *soul*.

And along the way, I want to free everyone I encounter from the fear of their own Greatness. I want to infuse them all with the raw courage it takes to hold nothing back, to drip-feed their minds with the singular belief:

I was created like none other.

I want everyone to see what I see: how magnificently we are made.

But even now, as I try to grasp this for myself, even as I see my own light within, I am in awe of the realization that I might be worthy of such a light. It just humbles me so…and it scares me. It scares me to think I might not have what it takes to achieve my Greatness. I might not pick the right dreams; I might take too many wrong turns in the pursuit of my life. And it makes me question…

If I become great, will I still be afraid? Do I really *want* to become great? And if I do, will they see too much of me and find me unworthy?

Will they expect me to *always* be great? And what would happen if I wasn't?

Would I feel their rejection? Would I feel their love only to have it taken away? Would I see disappointment in their eyes?

Regardless of all this questioning, in spite of my very real fears, I still have this insane desire to be seen—really seen. Hence the need to get up and go to work—unveiling who I really am and what's squirming around inside of me.

Make no mistake. I know that if I do the work, I will be seen—and not just in all my glory, but in all my nakedness as well. But I am older now; I don't think it scares me as much anymore.

So I will work every day. And my work is to get silent and *connect*— every piece of me, *all* the pieces of me—to my light, to the beacon of Life that is always there to guide me. Over the years, I have found that doing this work has enabled me to collect oodles of courage to help me surrender to all I can be.

And over time, doing this work has taught me to trust that I really do have a divine purpose. I may not have the slightest idea what it is and how it's supposed to manifest itself, but I do believe that Life will lead the way and the painting of my soul will reveal itself in good time.

Sometimes I feel so much peace and contentment in the entire process, it seems as if the clock stops ticking. Life becomes infinite and I am absorbed into Its *presence*, if only for a little while. Sometimes the pure Joy of experiencing my own soul just fills me to overflowing and I am called to share the abundance.

Like today, when I am on such a high. Today I am curious to see the effect of my Joy on those around me and I wonder:

Can they feel what I feel? Can they see all the way inside my soul right now?

If I sneeze hard enough, will they catch my Joy?

I guess the only way I will ever find out is to simply put myself out there.

So I will embark on this quest to be so bold as to shine my light for all to behold. I will sit back and watch what happens, as I am most anxious to be seen. My hope is that by experiencing the Joy within me, I might also set free the possibilities within others.

But it appears that today, I am to be disappointed.

It appears that today, I am not destined to help break any chains. I can't seem to break through the noise and busyness of their lives.

As I am searching for a response, as I am observing them to see if they notice me, I realize they aren't looking at me; I can't see my reflection in their eyes. For some reason, they aren't receiving the light I am sharing so freely with them. They can't feel my Joy, and I remain here unseen.

My Joy dissipates. They don't see me, and now I feel alone.

How did I get here? I was just feeling so alive.

I've realized, after sitting here mulling this over, that in my quest to reveal my Greatness, in my intention to share in the Joy of my aliveness, I may have taken a wrong turn.

Regardless of how amazing my Joy feels to me, and how eager I am to color my world with it, I have forgotten that—whether or not they see me—who I am and what my life is going to be about is inside of *me*, not *them*.

It seems *my fear of being insignificant has eclipsed my light.* And every time I look for *my* reflection in the wrong eyes, I can't see *me*.

It seems I have forgotten that my intention and my actions must be joined at the deepest part of me because they are partners in the revelation of my purpose. I have forgotten that it takes a great deal of *presence* to make sure a greatest *intention* precedes a desire to act in the greatest *good*. And I have forgotten I have other mirrors—other members of my Greater Power System that can reflect my Joy, reflect the art of *me*.

Regardless of the work I do to connect to my intention, today has shown me that it's not easy to restrain myself from searching for my reflection in the eyes of those few who can't reflect my Joy back to me, to set aside my need to witness their recognition of my worth. Today has shown me that it will take more work to remove the insecurities that are blocking my light. I will need to do my job to get out of the way of the *Greatness* flowing through me.

So now I will dive back into my work, connecting and trusting and fulfilling myself to overflowing again.

There is no loneliness here.

And as I work to get present within myself, I am reminded of my original intention:

I really just want to live, love, learn, and leave a legacy with Joy.

Once again, my Self reveals to me that it costs me nothing but my time and attention to rediscover who I really am. My time in the company of my own spirit reminds me that the Joy I experience is infinite, its life has no end; there's plenty more where it came from.

And I remember now: The light from this Joy comes *through* me, not *from* me. It is only mine to share, not possess. This Joy was designed to be given freely, with no expectations and no strings attached, except to be open to receiving more Joy from sharing it.

So today I will set out to purely spread a Joy virus.

I will spread the Joy I am experiencing as I unveil all the possibilities within me. I will find the consistent mirrors within my Greater Power System that I need to see my Self fully. I will share the Joy I am feeling as I shine all the Presence that comes through me.

And as I encounter those resistant souls, I will try to simply see— *really* see. Clear the lens of *my* mind, *my* beliefs, *my* judgments, and *my* fears, and just be present in their company…and reflect back to them all the beauty and truth that I know is there.

~

Author's note:

I have been called to teach. And I think every great teacher loves to see the look of understanding reach the eyes of those they teach. I know I absolutely love the feeling of penetrating someone else's world and seeing evidence that they now carry something new with them.

I believe I am a teacher at heart, but for the longest time, I had this dilemma…who and what was I to teach?

I had absolutely no training—other than what I learned in my own life.

So why was I being called to teach? *I didn't even know that much.*

All I knew was, the more I *thought* I knew, the more I needed to *learn*. And it was one thing to learn—we all learn; it was another thing to teach. Why was *I* being called to teach?

I wasn't anybody special. I wasn't anybody great. I was…nobody, really.

One day a few years ago, when I was feeling the clock ticking away in my life, I sat down to read through my journals. Even though I had reread them a thousand times, there was a time I saw something new.

I had discovered that whenever I held back from expressing my true Self, whenever I tried to either bury or discard a unique idea or a creative inspiration that was percolating inside of me, I felt invisible. And in contrast, whenever I leaked out to those closest to me some of the deepest, most authentic parts of me…whenever I was my most natural, most unreserved self…I felt *alive*.

When I started to connect the dots of my life, I discovered that I could feel great peace when I expressed myself creatively, and when the people around me found my creative work stirring and beautiful. I discovered that I could feel great Joy when I expressed my unique perspective, and when those that I shared it with found it inspiring and enlightening.

Something happened to me that day, and I finally woke up. I realized that I really didn't want to die with all this *life* inside of me… *unseen*.

So I surrendered. And I asked, "Why couldn't I teach just by expressing my real, authentic Self?"

So I released my unique perspective from the pages of my journals and liberated my creative Self from the recesses of my imagination. I now write books and paint art so that I can spend my life expressing my truth, my beauty…as seen through *my* eyes, heard through *my* ears, and felt with *my* heart.

The catalyst for this particular journal arrived when I was in the early stages of writing some of the other journals. Quite often, after I wrote what I felt was a very profound piece, one that spoke to me on a deep level, I would be moved to tears of Joy. I couldn't believe that what I wrote had come from inside *me*, and I couldn't wait to share it with my family and friends. I wanted their validation, their concurrence that what I had written was indeed as great as I felt it was. I was dying for their enthusiasm to match my own.

There were many occasions when I did receive their "applause," and it always felt great. But one day, after I had written one particular piece that had me really stoked, I was determined to share it with some of my family. With much anticipation, I sat them down and read my latest inspiration—but as I finished and looked up, I realized they weren't *there*. I could see the vacancy in their eyes; their minds were busy elsewhere. And I could see that I just couldn't penetrate their world with this *Joy* that I was about to *implode* in.

They responded with the perfunctory "That's nice" and went back to their previous tasks. I was left feeling dejected, deflated, thinking, How can I be so blown away by the beauty and truth of this, and they don't feel *any* of it?

I felt incredibly invisible. For a few days after that, I got really depressed and confused, and my joyful writing descended into:

Why am I doing this? I am being more real than ever and I'm *still* invisible. Am I crazy enough to think this work will resonate with *anyone*? *No one* is going to *get* me with this stuff. The world is too busy to *see* me.

I sat venting in my journal, pleading with my spirit to show me where I was meant to be, to show me what I was meant to do with my life, because clearly, *this* wasn't it. I was determined to give up all this work I had started and wait for my "real" Voice to lead me to where I was "really" supposed to be.

But after spending some time connecting to my Self, what remained in the silence…were the lingering memories, the persistent buzz from the Joy of how *great* it felt to create my art, and how *great* it felt to write these journals.

I realized then that my family didn't render me invalidated. I realized that, for whatever reason, they simply didn't see me that day.

And then I remembered the times when others *were* as moved as I was, when others *did* reciprocate my Joy. I remembered the times when I could *see* the change in them when I shared my work with them. I could *see* that they were carrying something new with them…and then I remembered how *significant* I felt when I was of service to *them.*

This "lack" of recognition—my failure to "teach"—became a profound reminder for me. It reminded me that I cannot become attached to a singular person's recognition of my beauty and truth. I must remain connected to my intention…and remember that *when the student is ready, the teacher will appear.*

And *this* student has learned that whether I succeed at this work with a particular person or not, it doesn't matter. Because the gratification comes from *doing* this work and being *one* with it. And with the right people, it just feels great to *share* it.

Yes, I hope the words will fly through the air to stick to them like bugs on a windshield. Yes, I hope the words will speak to them, move them, lift them, and comfort them. And yes, I would love to see evidence of this connection to their soul, see the recognition of its beauty and truth in their eyes…but in the end, what's most important is that this is the path I must take to feel whole and complete.

Ultimately, my intention is simply to unveil who I am. I could leave the words inside my journals, but for some reason, I am driven to release them from the pages of my privacy. I could create the art simply to decorate the walls of my own home, but I feel called to color my whole world with it.

If I release what lies deep within me with no strings attached, and this work speaks to them, great. If it doesn't, that's great, too. I have other mirrors. And I've already fulfilled a purpose. I am already complete in the *Joy*…of writing and teaching and painting, and then sharing it all. For now, this is how I express *my life's work.* Doing it deepens my life. And sharing it adds meaning and significance to it.

It is hard to write about my mission of teaching…it smacks of grandeur, not simple greatness. But I've made some progress with accepting this calling in me. I've started to make peace with this notion, because I don't view myself as a teacher; I view myself as a servant. Ultimately, I am *serving my soul*…and the Connection between *all* our souls.

It's taken me a long time to become this transparent. And it's not without fear. I bare my soul in spite of my fear, because I seek to be recognized as who I am. And I have come to the conclusion that this will never happen if I spend my life *hiding*.

It is a struggle to let go of the need for validation, to instead look within to find value in what I am doing, to use my own Voice to teach *me*…that I *am* indeed created like none other, I *do* have worth…and *I* am the one who needs to see it.

I still find that I don't want people to reject the deepest parts of me, to judge me unworthy; I don't want to be left alone. But if I concentrate on work solely so I can be visible, or if I build my life around work that is devoid of my passion and my Joy, or if I stray too far from who I truly am and what I am made of at the core, or if I don't surround myself with people who share my passion, I will feel empty, lost…*unfinished*.

In the end, it really doesn't matter what *work* I do: I just know I am *least alone* when I stay connected to the daily Joy that makes me feel whole and complete within a Greater Power System that consistently sees me.

I feel the most *recognized* when I connect to my divine light, when I unearth the deepest parts of my soul and its Joy rewards me for my efforts. I feel the most *seen* when the spotlight from my soul floods the stage of my life, blinding me in its truth and beauty, when my Greater Power System is in the audience cheering me on.

And the *Greatest presence* that I seek to radiate out into the world is most visible when I allow my light to shine its brightest and clearest—when I remain connected to my *Greatest intention.*

So I strip my spirit naked in the hopes that I can teach. I believe that when I express all that lies inside of me, I live as an example of the possibilities. And if I am an example of someone who is still standing when the divulging dust settles, then maybe that's how I will leave my mark.

When I write, my Greatness lies in the courage to lay this all out there—to be as honest and as open as I can, using my small, simple, ordinary life to help people not feel so alone. When I create, my Greatness lies in the fearlessness to reveal my interpretation of beauty—so I can use my small, simple, ordinary imagination to color the world with possibilities.

Within my transparency, within my authenticity, my intention is to produce a body of work that will inspire you to *your* Greatness. I strive to do this by connecting as deeply as I can to my *own* Greatness. I strive to just be the scribe and the painter…and *to get out of Its way.*

I believe we are all teachers. Everyone is here to teach something. I believe that within any common job or career, service or product, relationship or community, is the real work of embracing and sharing your exceptionality, your *un*commonness—which I also believe reveals *our oneness.*

I believe your real work is in releasing the universal beauty and truth that accumulates within *you*—so we can all learn, so we can all be inspired by *your* personal Greatness.

The Joy of Knowing

I have a very large family, most of whom are voracious learners, creators, and teachers, with positive, proactive, progressive attitudes and habits that finish the dreams they imagine and manifest, with Joy.

A lot of them are educated and have numerous self-taught abilities and strengths mastered, after acquiring and progressing transferable skills from training received in different jobs that they've done.

Many of them demonstrate patience with their persistent practice of learning and discerning necessary from unnecessary efforts to grow their Joy. They intentionally choose to grow their innate talents and skills, and, as a result, they have become masters of their crafts.

On the whole, they're a pretty joyful bunch—strong, wise, and passionate about their belief in doing the things that bring them the most satisfaction, while contributing to the Greater Good from within jobs they love and do immensely well.

So many of my family members are excellent models of living, loving, learning, and leaving a legacy with a positive, proactive, progressive mindset.

I was raised within a family culture of creative entrepreneurs who have astounding imagination. They use their imagination with talent and skill to manifest their successes, and then use their manifestations to grow their imagination to achieve even greater levels of satisfaction.

The culture of thinking that I grew up with was dominant with positive, proactive, progressive coaching in "Go ahead—do it, create it, build it, make it, learn it, try it," etc. We were comforted when they showed us how heavily invested they were in helping us to succeed.

They opened our eyes with what-if lines of questioning like, "What if you moved over here? What if you go over there, as an alternative? What if you look at it this way? What if you view it that way instead?"

They trained me with the Intuition Manual, with the Joy from knowing I experienced within their shared Joy offered to me over the entire course of my life, as they "raised" my spirit. And with the maturity of my spirit, I learned that I could acquire, maintain, and grow my power to imagine and manifest *more* Joy.

There is incredible power in being raised constantly by those whom we know have the skills, wisdom, and passion to lead us, in being raised proudly by those whom we know we can trust in the integrity of their word…and in being raised intimately by those whom we know can train us with *their* Joy, who train us with their Intuition Manual.

We all borrow from each other's trained intimate knowing of Joy, to strengthen our commitment to what we imagine for our Selves, to gut-check the ever-unfolding direction of progress within our dreams, and to lean on those who champion us as we finish our ever-greater dreams to our satisfaction.

My family is most insistent about our being trained in knowing Joy intimately. They are frequent cheerleaders with their statements of encouragement: "*I* know you can do it," and "Make sure *you* have fun," along with my personal favorites, "*I will help you*" and "*Let's do this together.*"

The Joy of Knowing

One of my nieces and I speak often about the Joy our family has when we're helping each other out with challenging tasks or creative endeavors.

I was raised in this environment where we strive to not perpetuate *bullsh-t*. We minimize the crap we encounter along the way because we know how to lift each other up and over it. We bypass the parts of tasks that stink with our laser intention on generating Joy that transcends the stress.

We seek to cultivate a constant *habit* of spreading the positive-thinking-fertilizer-stuff that others can grow their dreams in, especially during hardships.

When we work alongside each other, we focus on making the necessary chores fun by using our imagination. We pace our Selves all the way through to the finish line, according to the state of our Joy in our physical, emotional, mental, and social body.

We tell stories, make jokes, play music, boogie a little, sing some, talk through life's challenges, explore each other's ideas, take *enough* breaks, get fully engrossed in mastering the details and quality of the finish within our tasks, celebrate when we're done, and so on.

The chores cease to become chores to us—they just become tasks performed within the presence of each other's Joy.

I learned to make it a habit to weave as much of my imagination into my chores as I could, instead of waiting for the chores to get finished before I could have fun, until I was able to delegate or eliminate the chores I was physically, emotionally, mentally, or socially done with.

I used to make it a game to teach my kids to wash dishes when they were very young. When they were tall enough to reach the sink standing on a chair, I'd have them stand on the chair in front of me and take turns washing every dish with me.

They did this with me for *years*, never once viewing it as a chore.

For them, it was just playing with soapy bubbles, looking for the rainbows in them, learning the math of water in spoons vs. cups, having fun engaging in conversations with Mom, and getting satisfaction each time we put the last dish away together.

This would take extra time to do, but I was taught by my family that play wasn't just all at once at the end of a day, a workweek, or a career. Instead, play was constantly available to us via the imagination we embedded in the tasks we did all day long.

The key was whether we had the freedom of time and energy, and permission of power, to play with our imagination all the way through the completion of each task. This is what I endeavored to give my children as they were growing up.

The emphasis I had on exploring the art of *me* growing up became the single most important drive in me that continuously acquires, maintains, and *grows* the freedom and power to provide for, nurture, and protect the expression of *my* spirit, so I can lead by example.

Knowing this, I sought to teach my children to do tasks with as much freedom and permission to exercise their imagination as possible—washing the dirty dishes that they helped to make, included.

Tasks aren't neglected when imagination is allowed freedom and permission to co-create; they just include the satisfaction of a job well done, or they are delegated or not done at all if Joy is absent.

This frequently requires the inclusion of our Greater Power System to learn, then improve, and then master the knowing of what is necessary and not necessary for us to get our dreams done.

Being aware of when Joy rises in us gets both the right task and the *tasker...finished.*

Some of my family members and I can get insanely inventive and find new creative ways to take a repetitive, boring task and use our imagination to find Joy in it.

I remember as a child stacking firewood for the winter. Mom would start the base for me, and I was to place each piece of wood so that the wall of firewood would be balanced front to back and side to side so it wouldn't fall over.

At first, it was repetitively boring to me, but then I got into the challenge of "How neat can I stack it?" and "How well can I make the shapes fit together?"

I became fascinated with the grain and the bark, and the time would fly by as I was immersed in the "art" I was forming with my wood wall.

Art in all its forms is valued as hugely important in my family. We have artists in many disciplines. We have a real appreciation for the cellular fun we experience when we are able to express "the art of us."

We know each other's tastes and niches well, and we are constantly hitting each other up with ideas we come across that we know will get each other excited.

It took me a long time to realize that the emphasis from my family on the essentialness of pursuing the art of us, is something that has sustained my life incredibly—though it is not as much of a spiritual health priority for some people.

As I've said, when we do a task, we can get creative if it is paired with a different activity that engages our "art" senses while we complete the task.

For years, my mother requested that my brother Marcel mow the lawn, while also keeping all the wildflowers growing in patches across the yard left untouched. She wanted art to look at in addition to a vast manicured green lawn (aka, a repetitive visual to my mother.)

Every time the flowers were blooming, she had my brother mow the entire lawn in a crazy curlicue pattern, weaving in and around all the wildflower patches. (It made the resulting lawn look like the kids who came into my salon with butchered hair from their explorations of hairstyling with scissors that they had gotten ahold of.)

Bless my brother for the restraint he had in not denying my mother her Joy in looking at those flowers out her windows. (In her defense, Maine has some gorgeous wildflower species.)

We all still laugh at her adamant refusal to cut those wildflowers down until they were done blooming. But we were also used to the importance the family placed on seizing moments of Joy that add up to a life fully lived, and for my mother, the art of those flowers was not to be missed.

I, too, raised my children to engage with life from an artistic viewpoint—to augment the entire accumulation of tasks they needed to master all the way through adulthood with Joy that satisfies their soul.

My daughter learned knitting and crocheting at a young age. She was eleven when she started selling scarves at a number of Maine's many arts and crafts shows. And when she outgrew that as an adult, she transferred her skills to making gorgeous blankets.

To offset the repetition, she logs a zillion hours knitting and crocheting the blankets while sitting in family conversations, watching movies, or attending zoom meetings for her job.

The repetition of the movement of the needles in her hands is mostly by feel at this point, and she has honed her skill enough to add an accompanying activity that engages her. She gets to create gorgeous blankets while immersed in other activities with Joy.

Learning and then honing and mastering talents and skills takes a lot less time if we allow our imagination to exercise its desire to burn some calories for us by acquiring, maintaining, and growing our Joy within tasks.

My children were young when I started teaching them to practice experiencing Joy across all the different tasks there were to do around the home, in addition to washing dishes.

They *loved* doing "grown-up" stuff, so I tried to include them, as much as they were able, in learning how to do grown-up tasks.

At first, I started them out with very simple, small projects I picked out for them to learn baby steps in. Those projects grew the skills over time that later enabled them to tackle very large, complex projects that my children became completely at ease with.

Now they enjoy the high-quality completion of tasks they've mastered because they are easily navigated by their accumulated training.

One of those tasks was how to paint different items we had around the house. Bit by bit, I helped them progress their knowledge and skill in how to load their brush and roller, the angle to hold the brush, the pressure they needed to spread the paint with, the color wheel, the different kinds of paint, etc., as I oversaw their progress on one project after another.

Their skills grew over time with positive, proactive, progressive practice under step-by-step guidance, with a focus on the satisfaction of doing a job well and *receiving guidance in what that looks like.*

A continuous helping hand is essential to get results that satisfy. The spirit gets discouraged and gives up when we give someone a project and materials, but don't guide them step by step.

To get satisfaction across a lifetime, we must learn the full scope of what Joy is possible to attain, train in, and maintain.

Gaining skill requires patience on the teacher's part to allow the student's skills to grow, but also a commitment on the teacher's part to course-correct the student as they grow, so they don't spend a lifetime practicing doing something that doesn't bring them high-quality Joy.

Both my son and daughter can paint well and *know* they paint well. My daughter has frequently sought out painting jobs, and she paints her home and items in her home with great skill.

My son, Devryn, still does exceptional work as a residential and commercial building and vehicle painter as one of his jobs, which has evolved into remodeling both homes and vehicles. His skill at creating flawless finishes and his eye for design is just remarkable.

Both of my children have a well-trained eye in color and design, form, and function, and in *knowing* the satisfaction of a job well done, which they use as a transferable skill into their other jobs.

When we *know* what satisfaction feels likes at the level of the soul, *no one* can make us believe that it doesn't exist.

There isn't anything more sustainable to maintain our *knowing* than the repeated satisfaction of manifesting all that we imagine. It carries us through the barren times of missing freedom and blocked power.

I have a freedom from fear of the unknown, untested, and untried which was gifted to me from my family empowering me to manifest so much of my imagination.

When someone spends enough time and energy accumulating enough power and skill to maintain the knowing in their bones, they transfer all that power and skill to what they don't know…*yet.*

I do not let anyone else interfere with my listening to and following my GPS or try to make me doubt my knowing…that a Greater Power System is in my life providing for, nurturing, protecting me, delivering Joy to me constantly. No one gets to deface, rip out pages, or throw out the Intuition Manual.

Knowing that we know Joy intimately—that we know how to acquire Joy, maintain Joy, and grow Joy (no matter what anyone tries to make us believe otherwise)—helps us as we ride the spiritual river that carries us over and around any rocks that get in our way…like if someone's negative view of us or negative judgment of what we do attempts to make us believe that the art of us can't be done, shouldn't be done, or won't *ever* be done.

The knowing of what we *will* get done comes from having done some form of it in some capacity before. Knowing that the art of us *will* get done every step of the way is essential to getting anything *satisfying* done.

It is the will in our knowing that gets deeply developed within the practiced connection of our GPS, that gets carefully honed from within the Joy flowing inside us, that directs our actions.

Going about completing the art of us follows from our spirit continuously coaxing us, *willing* us, toward that which is necessary to get *our Selves* done.

And first on that list, that which our Greater Power System seeks to make sure *always* gets done, is our self-care.

While my childhood training included hitching Joy to necessary chores along the way to satisfying my Self with a manifestation, I was also trained to do what I could to eliminate unnecessary chores, as well as coached in how to get the *greatest* amount of Joy into my entire life every step of the way, not just at the finish line.

Hence my lifelong habit of guided journaling to help me spot the unnecessary chores and eradicate them from my life with the help of my GPS and grow the habits that bring me Joy and share that Joy within the Greater Good community.

Chores of physical labor, chores of mental labor, chores of emotional labor, chores of social labor are continuously honed down to the absolute minimum. With my GPS's help, the labor ceases to be painful.

I find I now perform labors of love that include Joy for me, instead. I wake up now realizing that I don't have the time or the energy to shovel bullsh-t.

I don't have the desire to use my time and energy here on earth to shovel any physical bullsh-t, emotional bullsh-t, mental bullsh-t, or social bullsh-t.

What I do have time and energy for are tasks that I can find a way to enjoy (even in the smallest amounts during *temporary* times), that positively proactively progressively connect me to me and connect me to others so I have all the tools at my disposal to manage my daily life to grow my time with Joy, and stop its being one lifelong "chore" to me.

The growth of Joy I experience when I do those tasks that I deem necessary to reach the finish line of my dreams enables me to fall asleep every night feeling blissfully *done*.

It's like I've just given birth...and I'm so overjoyed from the high I'm on from the realization of my dream. I'm holding in my arms the beauty and truth of what was once a possibility, now made real, and this makes all the "labor" *so* worth it.

I am awakened to the realization, to the knowing, that more Joy is now coming into my life daily, carrying me along toward more glorious destinations.

The birth of our dreams is like that of childbirth, but they can be birthed without the pain of labor. (Like the woman I knew in my salon who gave birth to six children with no labor pains. How cool.)

With birthing dreams, the labor "pains" that *I* choose to experience are the necessary efforts that give birth to the dreams that *I* desire. And I choose to refuse to labor at doing what causes me pain.

When I have consistent freedom to manifest my efforts—the labor "pains" aren't injurious, like they would be in an abusive environment.

When I am continuously free to go without sleep or miss a meal or make myself uncomfortable or sacrifice something temporarily in the ways *I* choose, I can make a wicked Olympic and efficient effort that has zero unnecessary chores or pain within it. I just have the thorough satisfaction of getting what I crave to finish, *done*.

My efforts don't subtract my Joy in any way, and they don't add stress in any form. Any intermittent "pains" are anesthetized with my impending Joy felt all along the way, culminating in a crescendo of satisfaction as I direct my physical, emotional, mental, and social body to contract and stretch my time and energy to birth all the results that I seek.

I believe we need to protect our freedom with choices that we know *we* can make, so we can maintain our knowing as best as we can, so we can exercise our Olympic efforts all the way through the finish lines, with dreams that have chosen *us*.

I protect my freedom when I use my knowing of what I can live with and what I can live without, to empower me to try all kinds of things, to master my self-care habits, and tweak all of my results.

I adjust my journey accordingly with Joy discerned from the directions I receive from my GPS. The *consistency* of Joy provides peace for me, nurtures me, protects me, from the fear of the unknown.

Training in incrementally challenging my Self to ever so slightly, over and over, stretch my capacity for Joy, and *not stress* until I reach my full, confident, comfort zone within a challenge, is crucial to me making love with life in freedom, completely.

I frequently teach my children and students that when we do something new, it's all unfamiliar. When we do it again in increments of full Joy, it's less scary because now Joy is becoming *familiar*.

Do it again, and now we can see our accrued skills and talents with Joy manifested, and we hitch our Joy to something new and unfamiliar, transferring what's unfamiliar into Joy that's now not so new or scary anymore.

Do this repeatedly, and we get into our Olympic effort zone. But it's *easy*, and not a grind—we go through life doing one "new" thing that we love after another, with just the right mix of confident comfort within a challenge that totally turns us on and keeps our Joy stoked all the way through—and once finished, satisfies us.

We go through life not saddling mistakes with shame, or sticking with what doesn't work out of fear. We just live, love, learn, and then leave our legacy.

I believe it's really just training our Selves to grow our time with Joy all the way through to the last breath we take here on earth.

If in the measure of your perfection
you feel inadequate with not giving enough,
and in the measure of your accomplishments
you are burdened with not doing enough,
perhaps in the measure of your life
you will realize you already are *enough.*

Wrap Us in the Gift of Your Presence

(One last journey through my journals...)

I am pausing to look at the woman in my reflection today...an unsure, questioning woman who is staring back at herself, thinking of all she is doing in her life, all that she is giving, and she is asking, "Is it enough?"

It's another day of contemplation, another moment of pause where she and I have stopped just long enough to agonize over how little we seem to have accomplished. To wrestle with the trying belief that our efforts will not produce any lasting effect or that we will not offer anything of significance in our service to the world.

We seem to have succumbed to our shortcomings—what we fail to have and what we have failed to give. And even as we reveal ourselves to the world, retreat inward to restore ourselves, and go back out to give more, we find we are on a perpetual treadmill of..."It's just not enough."

Even if we lead self-aware lives, even if we think deep down inside that we have something of value that's worthy of being unveiled, even when we know our intention is pure, when we tire, when we get busy, *we forget*.

We forget who we truly are and what we are truly capable of, and we immediately feel lacking. We think if we could rest more, we could do more. And if we could do more, we could be more, and if we could be more, one day we just might *arrive*.

But we never seem to get there. And we start to believe we are *simply not enough*.

And we ask, "How can we accept our limitations and ever *possibly* be enough?"

It appears we are people in the pursuit of some vague, unending, immeasurable achievement of perfection. And this pursuit is tough to let go of. It's nearly impossible to stop at *just enough*, to stop and not still feel the hunger, the insatiable need to be an infinite well of abundance. It seems that the incompleteness remains within, gnawing at our peace.

Why must it only be our *ideal* selves that are worthy of ever being enough? Why must the attainment of whatever it is we define as perfection be the yardstick by which we measure "enough"?

And I wonder, Will the day ever come when I will accept that I've done "enough"? Will the day ever come that will prove to me that I've *become* "enough"?

And the Voice speaks…

Well, in the interest of assisting you in the pursuit of your proof, I will reveal to you the truth.

Would you let me show you what I see? Would you let me share with you what I hear?

Would you consider that there are profound moments when you aren't looking, when you are unaware of your legacy that has been stamped on our hearts?

Could you open yourself up to the possibility that as you pass through our lives, no one else can touch us with their presence in the exact same way you can? And that when you leave the room, we can still feel the uniqueness of your character within your actions, continuing on within the impression you have left on our consciousness?

And did you know there is an intelligence in you that is unlike anyone else on this planet? And long after you have ceased speaking, we can still hear the distinct character of your thinking, lingering beyond the conversation, replaying in our memory like a tape?

And have you forgotten that no one else will ever look out at the world through your personal experiences, with your particular viewpoint…exactly as you do? That you could be halfway around the world, and we can still feel your presence, and in our minds we can still see your soul shining through those eyes.

You never know how you will impact someone else's life with your daily actions and thoughts and words; you never know how the simplest, most ordinary moment within your life could change someone forever.

You may not see it, but in those moments there is a seismic shift that your presence causes within us. These may be small, uneventful moments unnoticed by you, but they become great gifts that we now carry. These gifts penetrate us, rock our inner world, and become enduring parts of us. They become etched into our memory, and a permanent mark is made on our life.

Now you are in everything we do, in everything we give. It may be one single, precious moment that is a part of our past, but it will now continue to affect us, to teach us, because we all move forward by first looking back at where we have come from.

You must realize that there are profound milestones for us within the journey of your life, within the character of your love. You must realize, you give more than enough by being who you truly are—by becoming *more* of who you truly are and by sharing the journey to your Self along the way.

Being you is laced through everything you give and in everything you do. Being you is your single greatest gift to the world. And being you is the one thing no one else can do. Your greatest gift is being a real person with real fears and real dreams, who shows us real courage and real passion, and shares their real Self on their real journey.

You are as real as it gets…

…and it's more than enough.

You must take into consideration that it's within those moments of you being your most real Self that you leave your greatest mark, your legacy. You may have limitations in what you can do, and you may have borders to what you can give, but you have no end to who you are. You are not meant to one day present yourself as finished. You are never going to be finished.

It's time to abandon the pursuit of perfection. Perfection in the eyes of the real world is a fickle thing. Real perfection is actually *im*perfection, because it's within your imperfection that we can experience your true character. Your imperfection allows us to experience those unique pieces within you that peek through, revealing the quality of your soul.

There is perfection in the nicks and scratches of an entire life lived. Those rubbed-off spots are from many years of use—from you using your mind and your heart and your hands…to give and give and give.

Please know that you are seen, within your actions and within the intention of your heart, and that your life has not gone unrecognized. Your presence has taken up permanent residence in our minds, in our thoughts, and in our memories.

Your being has affected us…and we are altered.

So go ahead, rest…and know that you are enough.

Go ahead, smile…and know that you are loved.

~

Author's note:

This message was born in a conversation I had with my mother several months before she died. She had just woken up from a nap, and she invited me up onto her bed to talk. Aware that she was near the end of her life, we had many of these talks…profound, introspective, examining conversations. On this day, as I climbed onto the bed, she paused as if she was calculating how to say something. She took a breath and then just came out with it: "Anne, was I enough?"

I looked at her, ready to give a pat answer like "of course," but she stopped me and asked me again: "I want to know…did you get enough from me? Did I do enough? Was there anything missing from your life that you really needed from me?"

I lightheartedly said, "More piano lessons would have been cool." But then I realized the weight of her expectation; she wanted an *answer* and I really had to stop and think. Because I desperately wanted to give her the answer she wanted to hear.

And just as I was thinking that, she said, "Don't tell me what I want to hear, tell me the real truth."

Deeply respecting her request, I rolled onto my back, quiet. I lay there thinking back through my childhood…when I got my first job… when I got my first career…when I became a mother…all the way to this day on this bed. My life felt pretty amazing.

So I rolled back and was about to tell her so, but the look on her face struck me. This was more than the conventional question of "Was I a good enough mother to you?"; it was a much, much deeper need. This was the vulnerable face of "I want to know the answer…do you think I was a good enough *person*?"

I remember thinking at the time that this was ludicrous because through the years my mother had grown to be a consummate well of wisdom and support and a magnificent role model for how to become fully human. She was constantly reminding all of us younger family members how special we were, how precious we were. Never did I have an inkling during all the times I sat bathing in her encouragement and praise that this proud, strong, outrageously independent woman would not see her own profound value and *worth*.

It was then that my answer came: "No, Mom, you weren't enough—you were *more* than enough."

So if you are ever in doubt of your presence in this world, just look around at those who have left their mark on you. Do you think they realized a fraction of the power of their presence?

Have you told all the people who have ever left their imprint on your life that they still reside in you? Can you see the possibility that they might not realize the gift of their own presence?

Isn't it possible you might need to remember the power in your *own* presence? For it's possible that there are multitudes of minds and hearts carrying pieces of you around with them.

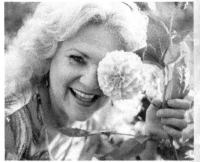
To sign up for *The Intuition Manual* online courses visit
www.hazelmariesgarden.com

~

Anne is a skilled teacher with the unique ability to tap into each student's strengths...as they progress [toward] being their most authentic and joyful self.
                                                    —Kim McClellan

~

[I took this class] to find more joy in my life and to be less stressed... and to focus on what is really important.
                                                    —Karen Montell

~

You, too, can transform your life through Anne's story and insights.
                                                    —Rev. Graham Connolly